Crusade to
Heal America

Crusade to Heal America

THE REMARKABLE LIFE
OF MARY LASKER

Judith L. Pearson

Mayo Clinic Press

MAYO CLINIC PRESS
200 First St. SW
Rochester, MN 55905
mcpress.mayoclinic.org

CRUSADE TO HEAL AMERICA: THE REMARKABLE LIFE OF MARY LASKER. Copyright © 2023 by Judith L. Pearson.

To stay informed about Mayo Clinic Press, please subscribe to our free e-newsletter at mcpress .mayoclinic.org or follow us on social media.

For bulk sales to employers, member groups and health-related companies, contact Mayo Clinic at SpecialSalesMayoBooks@mayo.edu.

Proceeds from the sale of every book benefit important medical research and education at Mayo Clinic.

Jacket design by Neill Fox, Foxnoggin.com

Library of Congress Cataloging in Publication data is available from the Library of Congress.

ISBN 979-8-88770-156-1 hardcover
ISBN 979-8-88770-157-8 ePub

Printed in Canada
First edition: 2023

For Kyla, Nicholas, and Charlotte: may you be inspired
by this portrait of courage and determination, and
may it embolden you to live your lives similarly.

Photo Credits

Prologue, Chapters 3, 4, 6, 7, 8, 12, 13 photos: Courtesy of the Lasker Foundation.

Chapter 1 photo: Courtesy of the Schlesinger Library, Harvard Radcliffe Institute.

Chapter 2 photo: Courtesy of the History Center of Lake Forest–Lake Bluff.

Chapters 5 and 16 photos: Courtesy of the Mary Lasker Papers, Rare Book & Manuscript Library, Columbia University in the City of New York.

Chapter 9 photo: "D1079–5a," *Omeka Experiment—Photos II,* accessed January 30, 2023, http://photos.lbjf.org/items/show/58558.

Chapter 10 photo: AP photo/John Lent.

Chapter 11 photo: Public domain.

Chapter 14 photo: Courtesy of Katrin DeBakey.

Chapters 15 and 17 photos: Courtesy of the Office of NIH History and Stetten Museum.

Epilogue photo: Courtesy of the author.

Contents

Author Note

In 1962, Columbia University asked Mary Lasker to record an oral history. She agreed, with the condition that it not be made public until after her death. The result was fifty-eight fabulous sessions, spanning two decades, and transcribed onto more than 2,100 pages. It is from this rich collection that I drew nearly all of Mary's activities, thoughts, and conversations included in this biography.

Mary's mother, Sara Woodard, also left behind a history in the form of a personal memoir, which Mary's sister, Alice Woodard Fordyce, typed up for posterity in 1989. Although it is not available to the public, it, too, provided rich insight into Mary's life.

Not wanting to distract from the story, I have chosen not to cite each time I used one of these sources. Rather, my hope is that you "hear" Mary's voice as clearly as I did. If you'd like to view the transcript of Mary's oral history, it is available free of charge at Columbia University Library's Oral History Research Office, under (appropriately) "Notable New Yorkers" (http://www.columbia.edu /cu/lweb/digital/collections/nny/laskerm/index.html).

Crusade to
Heal America

Prologue

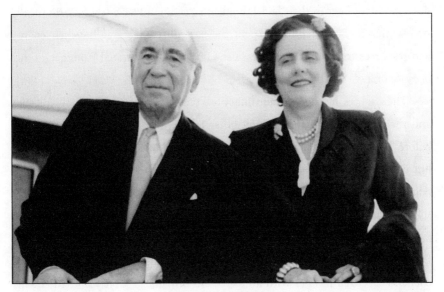

Albert and Mary on the deck of the Queen Mary *returning from Europe, circa 1948.*

The headline on the front page of the morning newspaper read: "Ike Turns Over NATO Command to Ridgway." General Dwight D. Eisenhower's May 31, 1952, move was made to pave the way for his presidential run (at which he succeeded in November of that year). But it was a headline below that would have far greater world impact: "Lasker, Pioneer in Advertising, Dies of Cancer."[1]

Albert Lasker had, indeed, been an advertising pioneer. But to reduce the sum total of his life to just that one accomplishment would be akin to mentioning that Leonardo da Vinci did a little sketching. And of all the journeys Albert had made in his seventy-two years, the most important one was down the aisle with his third wife, Mary Woodard Reinhardt.

Mary had not ventured far from her beloved husband since his diagnosis of "intestinal cancer" in his final months. She had been at his bedside on the misty morning he died in New York City's Columbia-Presbyterian Medical Center. Albert was Jewish, a faith whose tradition is to bury the deceased soon after death. Mary would follow through on the tradition, but first held a private funeral two days later in their lavish home on Beekman Place. It was sardonically surreal that a couple who had spent the past dozen years giving their energy and resources to conquer the disease should now be separated from each other because of it.

The Laskers had an extraordinary partnership. They were madly in love, and their marriage was unlike any other relationship either of them had had before. Each was successful in business, and each had strong personality traits, but like a beautiful mosaic, it all blended rather than conflicted. Mary guided Albert to appreciate fine art; he counseled her on how to garner publicity for their mutual passion, the cure of deadly and debilitating diseases.

Albert had built an immensely successful advertising empire, counting Lucky Strike cigarettes, Wrigley's gum, Sunkist oranges, and others among his clients. He retired in 1942 with an enormous amount of money and an equally enormous amount of time and energy needing a new direction. In December of that year, he and Mary launched the Albert and Mary Lasker Foundation to, as Mary described, "promote health through education and research." Their hope was that the small financial awards that followed would not only fund new research projects but also put those researchers into a brighter spotlight, potentially leading to further support. There was so much yet to be discovered.

At that time in America, heart disease, stroke, and cancer killed more people than all other causes of death combined. A heart attack or stroke was likely to end a life immediately, if not soon afterward. But cancer was by far the most feared, as it killed slowly, agonizingly. Patients languished in hospitals, their open sores emitting nauseating odors, their skin hanging loosely on unrecognizable faces, their screams of pain filling the corridors. Since most other horrific diseases were contagious, hushed questions about cancer's contagion abounded. Further whispers wondered if the patient had brought the disease on him- or herself through an illegal or immoral act. Such rumors and misinformation forced patients and their families into shamed isolation. Surgery, radium, and X-ray therapy made up the entirety of the era's treatment arsenal. Just one person in four would survive the diagnosis. Thus, with little at their disposal, doctors routinely avoided even disclosing the diagnosis of the "Big C" to their patients.

By the time of the Laskers' 1940 wedding, cancer was personal to each of them. Mary had watched close friends die of the disease; before they met, Albert's younger brother, Harry, had succumbed at the age of thirty-nine. A 1943 newspaper article prompted Mary to pay a visit to the American Society for the Control of Cancer. The staid organization, she learned, consisted of doctors and scientists whose sole focus was the treatment of the disease, not how to prevent or cure it. The society had a $50,000 annual budget (the equivalent of nearly $858,000 in 2023), with none of it earmarked for research. She made a $5,000 donation and went home determined to change things.

Together, the Laskers reimagined the organization, rechristening it as the American Cancer Society. With their help, and that of many well-heeled friends, the next year's donations were a whopping $4,292,000, with $960,000 designated for research ($72 million and $16 million, respectively, in 2023 dollars). It was a start, but Mary couldn't fathom why more institutions weren't involved in seeking a cure for the terrifying and deadly disease. Although they were fabulously rich, donating their own money, Albert explained, was not the solution. Rather, the United States government needed to be her target. He tutored her in the delicate nuances of fundraising for political candidates and "friend raising"— cultivating in those same politicians the Laskers' passion for medical research.

Mary was certainly not a politician, but she saw a clear path to blend Albert's lessons with her charming personality. The result became her ability to nudge the unconvinced, including scientists, doctors, members of Congress, and even presidents. She believed scientific research could save lives, even if the scientists didn't believe it themselves. Some of them would become friends; others would not be able to control their resentment at her success. But Mary truly didn't care. She was on a mission, creating an entirely new breed of citizen volunteer: the medical research lobbyist.

Joseph Stalin (who would die less than a year after Albert) is credited as having said about war, "The death of one man is a tragedy. The death of a million is a statistic." More than 220,000 Americans would die of cancer in 1952.[2] But for Mary Lasker, there was only one tragedy that year. Albert's death would propel her life's mission to slay the cancer dragon once and for all, saving millions far into the future.

Chapter 1

~

"New York Was the Place!"

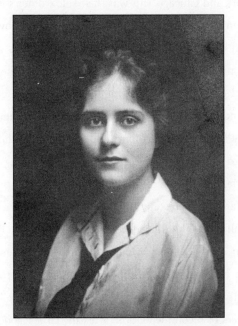

Mary as a student at Radcliffe, circa 1921.

The brick, limestone, and terra-cotta edifice rose twenty majestic stories above the corner of New York City's Lexington Avenue and 57th Street. Begun in 1920, with a final price tag of upward of $700,000 ($11 million today), this was more than an architectural gem in the heart of Manhattan.[1] The Allerton Hotel for Women was a luxurious combination of club and residence, built exclusively for the "New Woman." The term had been popularized at the end of the nineteenth century to define an emerging feminist ideal. Now, in the 1920s, the New Woman was here to stay, and not about to travel the customary path of the past, the one that led directly from her father's home to her husband's. Rather, she ditched her corset in favor of liberation, and let down her hair as part of a search for independence. The path she chose to travel took her out into the world—and, for those who were able, to New York City. It was the very path that led Mary Rae Woodard to the Allerton's front door in the autumn of 1923.

Although the hotel's parent company had built a number of exclusive men's hotels in New York and Chicago, this was their sole women's iteration, and it offered distinctly feminine features. Walking into the main lobby from 57th Street, Mary was greeted every day with a display of fresh flowers on the front desk. The "visiting salons" opening off the lobby ensured that "the occupied woman can entertain and enjoy the privileges of social life as she could at home." A large restaurant and offices filled out the rest of the ground floor. An elegant and gracefully curving stairway led residents and guests up to the mezzanine, with its balcony open to the lobby. Here there were larger drawing rooms, and above that was a cafeteria, from which tasty meals could be had at prices far below the cost in most of Manhattan's restaurants. Those were, however, the only spaces in which men were allowed. The Allerton's director, Miss Grace B. Drake, saw to it that the remaining eighteen floors belonged exclusively to the women.[2]

The Allerton had opened on October 16, 1922, filled to capacity, with a lengthy waiting list. Nonetheless, nearly a year later, Mary had produced the requisite two letters of recommendation, attesting to her good and moral character, and secured a room. Whether arranged as small suites or eight-by-ten-foot individual rooms (as Mary's was), each of the 448 living spaces had certain elements in common. They were cleverly furnished with pieces deliberately crafted on a smaller scale. The narrow, single beds had no footboard and a low headboard. The desk and chest of drawers were also petite, as were the chairs. Thus, although providing "unusually refined surroundings," the furniture's size gave the rooms a feel of being larger than they actually were.

The wall colors, bed linens, floor coverings, and draperies were all tastefully coordinated. And each room was equipped with the modern necessities of running water, electricity, and telephone. In place of the showers offered at the men's hotels, the women had baths. The closets were larger, the better to accommodate a working woman's wardrobe. And should that wardrobe need augmenting, the hotel provided a shopping service. Mary could also avail herself of the in-house bookstore, beauty salon, and laundry and seamstress services. The Allerton's crowning glory was at its crown: the rooftop. From the skyscraping garden, solarium, and large ballroom, Mary could look down upon Central Park and the gilded mansions of "Millionaire's Row" along Fifth Avenue.[3]

Miss Drake had said in a newspaper interview that the Allerton was "a haven which . . . include[s] a note of beauty which means so much to the woman of education and refined tastes."[4] That was an apt description of twenty-two-year-old Mary. Armed with drive and a plan, she was certain New York—and the Allerton—"was the place" for her to begin her career, she later said. Plus, Mary Woodard had an ace up her sleeve. She had been prepared for this important first step into adult life by the perfect role model. A generation earlier, her mother, Sara, had traveled a very similar path.

⟿

Sara Johnson had lived the entirety of her eighteen years in Portadown, Ireland's linen capital. Now, on a sunny day in August 1880, she stood on a pier in Queenstown, 250 miles from home, about to begin a journey to America. Sara loved Ireland; she loved her life. But it was not a quiet one. Her father, a successful linen merchant, had married three times. His first two wives had produced a total of six children before dying. His third wife had given birth to five more, including Sara. That kind of scenario wasn't in Sara's immediate plan. She hoped to find a different life in London, Ontario, at the end of the forthcoming journey. There she would live with her brother, a successful dry goods merchant.

Eight days after leaving Queenstown, the ship slipped past the Statue of Liberty at 11:00 p.m. The next morning, Sara, along with the other immigrants aboard, was carefully registered, and she picked up her luggage. She spent two days taking in the city's sights before catching a train heading north. Sara's Canadian stay, however, was short; helping to care for her brother's children wasn't much different from being home in Ireland. Her half-sister lived in Chicago, and that exciting and growing city now called to her.

With her brother-in-law's help, she secured an interview at the prestigious Gossage and Co. department store. Charles Gossage himself interviewed her, asking if she had sales experience. She told him she had none but added that someone had to give her a chance so she could gain experience. Gossage was impressed and hired her. Not long afterward Gossage died suddenly, and the store was sold to Carson, Pirie, Scott and Co.

At the time there was no such thing as "ready-to-wear" in women's clothing. Rather, all stores employed dressmakers, each building their own clientele. When an opening as manager of the entire dressmaking department became available, Sara got the job. Soon she was managing a staff of over a hundred and was responsible for more than $100,000 in annual sales (the equivalent of more than $3 million today). She took head dressmakers to Paris in search of the latest styles, prompting a newspaper writer to say that her "wit and will" had made her one of the highest-paid women in Chicago. She moved into a lovely apartment building located near the store and became close friends with fellow boarders Angie Fellows and her doctor husband.

In May 1893 the city buzzed with excitement as the World's Columbian Exhibition opened. Locally referred to as "the fair," it spanned Chicago's lakefront, celebrating the four-hundredth anniversary of Columbus arriving in the New World. The fair debuted a new attraction, the Ferris wheel, bringing millions from around the world to ride it, including Angie's cousin Frank. The handsome, soft-spoken bachelor banker from Watertown, Wisconsin, had no idea his excursion to the city would result in such important consequences for his life. Neither did Sara when she accepted Angie's invitation for dinner while Frank was in town. After that introduction, Frank and Sara corresponded, and visited back and forth between Watertown, near Milwaukee, and Chicago, 150 miles south. Attraction became friendship, and friendship became love. The two were married at the Fellowses' new home in March 1897, and after a wedding trip they settled in Watertown.

Although he was a quiet man, Frank Woodard was one of the most respected—and financially successful—individuals in town. In addition to his position at the bank, he, too, had an entrepreneurial spirit and had invested in a number of lucrative businesses. That paved the way for the Woodards to build one of the most beautiful houses in Watertown. The large, three-story house was surrounded by gardens and lawns. Cream brick framed tall windows on the first two floors, which boasted four bedrooms and two bathrooms (quite a luxury for the time).

Sara's business days might have been over, but she found plenty to occupy her time. Missing the beauty of Ireland, she threw herself into city beautification. It wasn't a question of Watertown not being pleasant. For Sara, there were never enough flowers, which led to the opening of two new city parks. Education—formal or otherwise—was important to her, too. Most men, and nearly all women, did not seek higher education. Some never even left Watertown. But they could travel the world through books, so Sara set about having a municipal library built, thanks to a grant from industrialist Andrew Carnegie's foundation.

The musical society and the women's club at the Congregational Church served to satisfy Sara's drive to lift women to the heights they desired. She never accepted no as a response to something she sought; she simply went a different route to get to yes, whether it was from Frank or the city council. Her focus was laser sharp in all of these ventures until the day after Thanksgiving, 1899. That was the day Mary Rae Woodard came into the world.

Beautiful and precocious, Mary was the center of attention no matter where Sara and Frank took her. When she was nearly five, Mary made it known she was ready for a little sister, and *only* a sister. She included the request in her prayers until it was answered in 1906, when Alice was born. Mary's cousin relayed that he, too, had prayed for a little sister but hadn't gotten one. Mary informed him, "You didn't pray hard enough."

There was never a question in Sara Woodard's mind that her daughters wouldn't receive the best education, no matter the cost. Therefore, after grammar school in Watertown, Mary was enrolled at a boarding school in Madison, forty miles away. There she met Pauline Pabst. The granddaughter of a Great Lakes shipping magnate whose fortune was augmented in the brewing industry, Pauline was full of fun. With five siblings, the Pabst home was always lively, and Pauline carried that enthusiasm for life wherever she went. The girls were inseparable, so when Pauline decided to attend the University of Wisconsin in 1918, Mary followed her.

Free from parental and boarding school oversight, Mary dove into parties and what she would later call "running around with boys." A suitor interested in a date had to wait three weeks for a night to open up. She was keen to be a good student as well, juggling her social life with late-night study sessions. But while rushing the Delta Gamma sorority, she began to feel ill and nearly collapsed. She was diagnosed at the campus infirmary with Spanish flu, the influenza that was spreading across the world.

The flu was just one serious illness in what seemed to Mary like a very long chain of them. Every winter, as a small child, she had been plagued by "mastoids," the era's term for a condition now known as mastoiditis. Usually induced by an untreated acute middle ear infection, it was a leading cause of child mortality until antibiotics came onto the scene. One year Mary's case was so severe that she later recalled awakening from a feverish sleep, with her mother sitting beside her bed and a friend hovering behind. "Oh Sara," the friend said, "I don't think you'll ever raise her." Even at that young age, Mary remembered feeling that the woman had made a mistake in her judgment. Death was *not* in her near future.

With regular diagnoses of dysentery and anemia following her through childhood and into young adulthood, Mary's frustration with illness grew. At the time of her flu diagnosis, she was kept in quarantine with dozens of others, lined up in rows of cots, many more ill than she was. There was no cure, and the treatment was limited to Argyrol (an antiseptic containing a compound of silver and protein), which was liberally administered. Mary realized she and her fellow patients were helpless, and she made a resolution: "If the time ever comes, I am going to do something about finding new knowledge against disease, and see to it that medical education is improved."

Once Mary had recovered from the flu, Sara had no intention of allowing her to return to the university social life that had so worn her out. She needn't have worried; Mary had already decided her future lay in the art world. The only college offering an art history major was Radcliffe College in Cambridge, Massachusetts, and off she went. While her personality was still a magnet for new friends, her studies were so intriguing, they took precedence over her social calendar. Personal causes, however, were another story.

When she found that her dormitory had neither dining room curtains nor a full-length mirror, Mary took up a collection and had both installed. When spring arrived, the prom committee announced it had hired Leo Reisman and his newly formed band to play. Mary knew he was a hot commodity, and so she persuaded the committee to boost the price of tickets, thus enlarging the class coffers. Although she'd had a number of beaux at Radcliffe, her prom date was a special Harvard man. They routinely spent time together on a park bench, eating brownies he'd received from home. But in the end, Mary didn't think he was ambitious enough, and the romance never flourished. She wanted to love and be loved, but she also had a desire to do the best she could in life, even in love.

She graduated from Radcliffe cum laude with a degree in art, and then did a semester of postgraduate work at Oxford. When it was over, Sara and Alice arrived, and the three women spent the summer in France, giving Mary an up-close examination of the art she'd only just read about. By summer's end, her career path was certain: she would become a successful dealer in the heart of America's art world.

As she had done every weekday morning since her October arrival in New York, Mary left the Allerton Hotel, walked three blocks west to Fifth Avenue, and headed south. She walked past the Knoedler Gallery, which had been her first destination upon arriving in the city. A much-loved Radcliffe professor had given her a letter of introduction to Roland Knoedler, owner of the renowned art establishment. He didn't have a position for her but recommended she visit Mr. Harold Ehrich on the next block, who hired her on the spot.

The gallery specialized in the works of old masters, artists who were fully trained and painting in Europe before the 1800s: Hals, van Dyck, Rembrandt, Gainsborough, and Rubens, among them. These were not, unfortunately, what Mary would be selling. The gallery also had a collection of china, glass, and small objets d'art. It was those Mary was to sell, working solely on commission, and earning a paltry $9 a week. But it was a job. And in New York, having a job was what would lead you to the next one, and hopefully a step up. As her mother had learned before her, when it came to selling, it was all about experience and getting that first big break.

It was a fabulous time to be a New Woman in that vibrant city. And Mary certainly fit that description, wearing the latest fashions: straight lines, a dropped, loose waist, and a considerable amount of leg showing below the knee. Even the shoes showed skin, as opposed to the buttoned-up version the older generation still wore. The New Woman was liberated socially as well. She could vote, smoke, and, if she wanted to, enter any one of the many speakeasies that had cropped up around the city since Prohibition was declared in January 1920. It wasn't long before Mary met another New Woman with similar roots and a similar zest for life.

Born in a small Indiana town shortly after Mary, Eleanor Lambert also had big dreams. Eleanor's specialty was publicity, with a goal of representing art dealers. She and Mary had crossed paths at a party. An instant—and lifelong—friendship developed. In an effort to further both of their careers, they conceived the idea of a weekend art exhibition, proceeds from which would go to charity.

They persuaded an imperious gallery owner to loan them space, and then visited other galleries, pressing them into loaning paintings for their show. At Durand-Ruel, another starchy gallery, they informed the owner he was rumored to possess Renoir's *La Tasse de Chocolat* (*Cup of Chocolate*). Could they borrow it? He was both angry and amused, and led them upstairs to view the famed painting. They harassed him until he agreed to loan it to their good cause. To the dealer's amazement (and the girls' good fortune), Edsel Ford strolled into their exhibition and bought the Renoir for $125,000 (over $2 million today).

Not long after, Knoedler invited Mary to stop by his office on her way to work. There he introduced her to Paul Reinhardt, the thirty-four-year-old owner of a gallery that also specialized in old masters. Reinhardt's father, Henry, had opened it in 1911, and when he died unexpectedly ten years later, Paul had taken over. Now he was looking to hire someone to run exhibitions for him. Mary impressed him, and by the dawn of 1924 she was working for him.

Reinhardt was a widower, and, as Mary later described, she found him "to be very pleasant with a great feeling for art." At a time when all things Spanish were in vogue, she convinced him to hold an Ignacio Zuloaga exhibition. Zuloaga was the best-known contemporary foreign artist at the time. His paintings had been to the United States, but the artist never had until January 4, 1925, when he arrived for the opening reception at Reinhardt's gallery. The show was described in the newspaper as a retrospective, including some of his older pieces, plus special favorites never before exhibited in America. All had a Spanish motif, of course, including "toreadors, Spanish dancers, portraits of American and Spanish social celebrities, and landscapes." As the article continued, "It is life, stark or sophisticated, which Zuloaga paints."

The show continued until the end of the month, and the dramatic exhibition attracted more than eighty thousand visitors, bringing in nearly $250,000 in sales.[5] It accomplished two more, equally important things. First, Paul realized that his new associate was as smart as she was attractive. And second, he felt himself falling in love with her.

Paul Reinhardt had been born into art in Chicago in 1889. By the time he was nineteen, he knew the old masters well enough to begin his career in the family business. On a buying trip to New York a year later, Paul not only gleaned a new Rubens for the Reinhardt inventory but also met Clara Baumgarten. The two were married in January 1911, and shortly after, Paul and Henry moved their gallery from Chicago to Fifth Avenue in New York City.

Henry made Paul an official partner in the firm, and Reinhardt and Son climbed to significance in the art world. Life was good until Clara died in 1923. When Paul hired Mary a year later, she was a breath of fresh air in his now empty life. She was young and vivacious, and excited to apply her knowledge about art and artists. She was also the only art dealer in the city (man or woman) with a degree in art history. While Mary respected the old masters, which had been the gallery's bread and butter, Paul began to realize that "modern" art could also be lucrative. After their successful Zuloaga show, Mary began singing the praises of little-known French impressionist Marc Chagall. She persuaded Paul to host Chagall's first American exhibition in January 1926. But her earlier success with Zuloaga was not to be repeated. "[Chagall] was unknown and totally crazy," she later said. "Not one single thing was sold."

That, however, did not cool Paul's love for Mary. He had proposed the previous year, but there was a problem. Paul Reinhardt drank too much. Sara had told her daughters stories of a brother, who, according to Sara, had "ruined his family because he was an alcoholic." Mary had no intention of experiencing that kind of disgrace. She told Paul that she'd marry him if he stopped drinking. "I'll give it up," he proclaimed. She was skeptical, but he remained dry for a year. So on May 23, 1926, Mary became Mrs. Paul Reinhardt. She was twenty-six, he was thirty-seven.

The newlyweds spent their honeymoon in Europe, which doubled as a buying expedition. Mary was fascinated by impressionism. Van Gogh, Picasso, Renoir, Matisse, Braque, and Utrillo were all exciting, and she could see they were the future in art. The Reinhardts came home with bundles of them, picking up fresh canvases for a song. They bought several watercolors by Raoul Dufy for $70 or $80 each. (Those same paintings sell for nearly a thousand times that today.) Mary held back some of their purchases as a foundation for a personal collection. The others they arranged among the more traditional pieces in the gallery, mixing Rembrandt and Renoir, Titian and Picasso.

Their life was pleasant. At a time when steak was 26¢ a pound, their gallery was grossing $500,000 annually. They were well known and well respected around New York, attending galas and events of every kind. They repeated their European trek each summer and created a clientele that thought nothing of spending tens or even hundreds of thousands of dollars in just one visit. After all, the Roaring Twenties continued to roar, with the Dow Jones average reaching a peak it wouldn't achieve again for thirty-five years.

Then, on October 29, 1929, it was all over. The stock market collapsed, with over sixteen million shares changing ownership in just that one day. Billions of dollars were lost, and thousands of investors were bankrupted. By the following day, the panic selling had reached such a peak that some stocks couldn't find buyers at any price. American financial giants like the Rockefellers, William Durant, and others tried to shore up confidence in the market by buying huge amounts of the nearly worthless paper. But it was too late.

As the days and weeks passed, some of those who had been the most heavily invested couldn't bear the pain of losing everything. Across New York and around the country, they set themselves on fire, inhaled automobile exhaust, or jumped from high-rises. Things were bad for the Reinhardts, too. Even though many of the gallery's clients were still very rich, they lay low, either out of sympathy for those who'd lost everything or out of fear of being robbed. Paul seemed surprised by this; he had expected to continue to make big sales to them. And instead of considering what other business he might go into or what else he could do, he just told Mary, "Well, I'll wait until this passes by." And while he was waiting, he started to drink again, sinking into severe alcoholism. "His anxiety was overwhelming and he became another person," Mary described. "It was as if he had retreated into a cave out of which you couldn't bring him or even reach him."

There was no general knowledge of what to do for alcoholics in those years. Alcoholics Anonymous would not be founded until 1935, and it would be another four years before its famous "Twelve Steps" were published. A few times, when Paul was so incoherent Mary thought he might die, she put him in the hospital. He was given large doses of B vitamins, which certainly helped his poor nutritional state, but it did nothing to decrease the drinking. It would be decades before any drugs were developed to aid in alcoholics' recovery.

Several years earlier, Mary had become intensely interested in the new subject of psychoanalysis. Sigmund Freud had founded the clinical method, which used dialogue between a patient and a psychoanalyst to arrive at solutions for the patient's problems. Mary had read excerpts from Freud's collection of lectures, *Introduction to Psychoanalysis*. She had enthusiastically encouraged Paul to read some of the book as well, not because she thought he needed analyzing (he was not drinking at that time) but because she was intrigued and wanted to share it with him. His reaction to the material, however, was not one of interest but rather extreme shock, fear, and distress. Mary assumed it must have touched on some unknown neurosis that she didn't understand.

Yet, in an effort to help him when the world's ever-increasing financial struggles began closing in, Mary got him to agree to see a psychoanalyst. When he came back from his first appointment, she asked him, "Well, when are you going back again?" He replied, "I don't have to go back," to which she inquired, "Why not?" His answer: "I've been analyzed. That's it." But that couldn't be "it" for Mary.

⟶

Of course, Mary's interest in the mysteries of the mind wasn't unique in the world. Swiss psychiatrist Adolf Meyer was a contemporary of Sigmund Freud. Meyer found many of Freud's ideas and methods insightful. But he rejected psychoanalysis in favor of his own theory, which wove together biological, social, and psychological factors and symptoms to explain mental disorders. He called it "psychobiology." Neither man, however, was alone in trying to uncover the origins and treatments of mental disorders.

As was the case with many diseases and health conditions in previous centuries, mental illness was first thought to be the result of demonic possession or retribution for sins, and treatments were often barbaric and inhumane. Practitioners drilled into patients' heads to release evil spirits. With the advent of electricity, shock therapy, too, was attempted to bring patients back to "normal." Doctors also turned to lobotomy, a surgery that removed what was thought to be the problematic part of the brain. In the end, the step most families and legal authorities took was to house the mentally ill—a classification often including alcoholics and the homeless—in hospitals and asylums, out of the way and out of sight.

Most of the era's asylum residents were institutionalized either against their will or without understanding their plight. Often they lived in filth; some were chained to the walls or their beds. The doctors and attendants believed the common myths alleging that those with "abnormal" mentalities were unable to reason or control themselves, were capable of violence without provocation, didn't feel pain or temperature as "normal" people did, and could live in miserable conditions without complaint.

By the time Meyer arrived in the United States in 1892, he had already witnessed similar conditions in asylums in Europe. Such maltreatment sickened him, and he resolved to find better and much more humane ways to help patients. In further developing his psychobiology approach, he decided that, rather than focusing on mental "illness," he would focus on mental "hygiene" (hygiene being the process by which one achieved health, whether physical or mental). Meyer's work was highly respected and very well known.[6]

One day in 1907, Clifford Beers walked into Meyer's office. Beers had suffered a breakdown and made a half-hearted suicide attempt. He had been institutionalized, and experienced the inhumane treatment so common at the time. He was far more lucid than his fellow patients, however, and wrote *A Mind That Found Itself*, the saga of his odyssey in the asylum. Beers had come to Meyer with two goals. The first was for Meyer to review his eighty-thousand-word manuscript. That manuscript, he hoped, would play a role in his second goal: much-needed institutional reform.

The highly esteemed Meyer was intrigued and excited to meet Beers. The two men exchanged almost daily letters and express packages with ideas and rewrites until the book was finally published in 1908. The immediate result was public support for the mental hygiene movement. In 1910, Beers, Meyer, and others launched the National Committee on Mental Hygiene, with Meyer as chairman and Beers as executive secretary. The committee and the mental hygiene movement would continue to grow, eventually coming to Mary's attention decades later.

⟋

As the Depression continued, Paul Reinhardt was either unable or unwilling to quit drinking, and Mary was at her wits' end. Furthermore, both the gallery's and their personal financial positions were precarious. Covering the upcoming "season" in her August 30, 1931, column, New York art critic Lillian Semons remarked that most galleries were not commenting on their plans. However, Semons wrote, "Mr. Reinhardt will soon be on his way to Paris for a short time and he expects to return with a generous load of prizes from the studios there." Mrs. Reinhardt was apparently staying home.[7]

Semons noted that in their first show that season, "there will be paintings by Hals, Rubens, Van Dyke, . . . Redon, Renoir, Degas and others. Bringing the show up to the present will be paintings by Picasso and probably Utrillo. For the most part, the paintings are now in the private Reinhardt collection."

Translation: the Reinhardts would be selling some of their own art to stay afloat. Mary later said, "He [Paul] and I made a small collection of contemporary French pictures, paintings by Picasso, Matisse, Modigliani, Sutien, and maybe a couple of others. . . . I actually sold these pictures because we were hard up. The pictures had already gone up somewhat in value and I sold them at profit. I still regret selling some of them."

Finally, in 1932, Mary realized sadly, "I never could get him back. I was absolutely in despair. I couldn't get him to stop drinking, I couldn't get him to do anything. I finally decided that I couldn't survive myself any longer . . . if I were to continue to be so frustrated." Mary left the gallery and moved out of their home.

Now came the question of how she would survive financially. She had recently become aware of the existence of chain stores. Possessing the entrepreneurial spirit her mother had, Mary was thrilled by the concept that you could meet with just a few buyers from a chain, and your product would then appear in all of their stores across the country. At the same time, she discovered Hollywood and the movies. Science fiction thrillers *King Kong* and *The Invisible Man* and comedies like Mae West's *She Done Him Wrong* and the Marx Brothers' *Duck Soup* were all hits that year. Irene Dunne, Ginger Rogers, and Fay Wray pranced across the screen in all their beauty and finery. And Mary got an idea.

Movies were an escape from the gloom of the Depression. But there was nowhere to find information on favorite stars or directors. Why not, she asked her friend Mary McSweeney, create a movie magazine? Something produced on slick paper with intelligent writing. The two women spent months on the idea. Mary took their plan to an advertising agency, seeking advice. The man she met with said her movie magazine wasn't a good idea. He advised her to do something with fashions or dress patterns, and another idea was born. Mary McSweeney's husband worked for the publisher Condé Nast, which produced Vogue dress patterns, and facilitated a meeting with the head of Vogue.

Money was still tight in most households, the two Marys explained, and many women had turned to making their own clothing. They proposed a line of patterns to be called Hollywood Patterns, each featuring a photo of a famous female movie star. It would make their patterns stand out from the others. And their clientele would feel they were wearing the same glamorous dresses their favorite stars wore, rather than something homemade. At the last minute, Mary McSweeney backed out of the business, but Vogue was on board. With releases from the various movie studios, they went into production. Mary sold the patterns to chain stores at a retail price of 15¢. She received a royalty of one-third of a cent on every pattern sold. The enterprise had a slow start. The official first day of sales was March 6, 1933, the same day President Franklin Roosevelt closed the banks for a week in response to a month-long run on them. But with ads that proclaimed "Hitch your fashion to a star!" and "Inspired by favorite screen stars!" Mary stayed the course. It wasn't long before women were catching Hollywood fever and stores from coast to coast were selling Hollywood Patterns.

The high of that success was deflated five months later. On August 2, around noon, Mary's father, Frank, was in a meeting at city hall in Watertown when he collapsed. As soon as Frank was brought home and Sara saw him, she knew he'd had a stroke. The right side of his face was completely paralyzed. He died two hours later, at the age of seventy-six. Mary had had a complicated relationship with her father. She loved him dearly, but his penny-pinching control over anything Sara wanted to purchase (never a frivolous request) made Mary vow she would always have her own money. Ironically, in planning his estate, Frank had seen to it that she would, indeed, be free of financial woes. He provided amply for her, as well as for her mother and sister. Mary took on the role of family money manager, overseeing the finances of all three of them.

Perhaps it was this recognition of the fragility of life that caused Mary to finally close her Reinhardt chapter. Ironically, her good friend Kay Swift, a successful music composer, was in a divorce frame of mind as well. Mary had met Kay when she first arrived in New York. They were so close, in fact, that Kay was generous with her designer clothes and previous years' mink coats. Mary had gotten to know Kay's family as well, and was heartbroken when Kay's mother, Ellen Dorr, died of breast cancer in 1928.

Kay had increasingly been seen around New York with George Gershwin. Inconveniently, she had also been married for sixteen years, much of it unhappily. The two women traveled to Reno, Nevada, where their divorces were finalized on December 20, 1934, at the Second Judicial District Court. Afterward, they took the two-minute walk to the Virginia Street Bridge spanning the Truckee River. Following tradition, they stood with their backs to the river, held their wedding rings in their right hands, and threw them over their left shoulders into the water below. Surely better things would be ahead in the new year.

Chapter 2

～

"That Man Is Making
a Great Mistake"

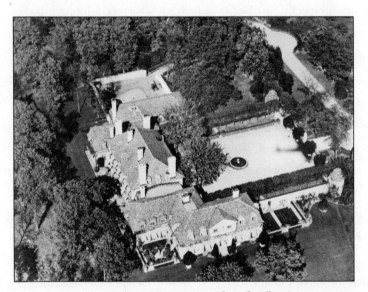

Aerial view of Mill Road Farm, circa 1926.

Albert Lasker was twenty years old and living in Chicago when a
tremendously powerful hurricane struck his hometown, Galveston, Texas, in 1898. It killed more than forty-two hundred citizens
and washed away a great deal of the city. His father, Morris, a successful and
well-respected Galveston businessman, stepped up to head the recovery and re-
building efforts. He was exceptionally community-minded, already donating to
the public schools, a local orphanage, and—being Jewish, albeit not particularly

observant—an institution that trained Jewish immigrants escaping the Russian pogroms. The influence of Morris's generous heart and spirit would guide the younger Lasker the rest of his life.

The letters Morris sent to Albert detailed the hurricane and its destruction. But Albert was about to launch a storm of his own. Before he left Texas, Morris had connected his son with Daniel Lord, a managing partner of the Chicago advertising firm Lord and Thomas. Father promised son that if advertising, a respected industry, didn't work out, Albert could return to his first love, journalism—a less respected avenue.[1]

Lord and Thomas was headquartered at the bustling corner of Wabash and Randolph (ironically, just blocks away from where Sara Johnson had worked a few years earlier). Albert loved the pulse of the city, even if he didn't relish his job. Advertising in that age was all print, and primarily in newspapers. The ads had no photos, no graphics of any kind, and the accompanying copy was often long and drab. Albert hated his job, but he was tethered to the agency because of a $500 gambling debt he had incurred in a craps game.[2] Albert was terrified of the game's organizer, a shady and threatening fellow. He had no savings and $500 was one-third of his annual salary. He had no choice but to plead his case to the firm's other partner, Ambrose Thomas, who took pity on the young man and gave him a loan to cover his debt. Albert was to be, essentially, an indentured servant until it was paid off, so he plowed forward.

Amazingly, he stumbled from one success to another. He landed new business and increased the advertising budgets of current clients. He discovered that he had a talent that many other early admen lacked: the ability and willingness to sell, first himself and his firm to the client, and then the client's products or services to the public. And along the way, Albert sold his superiors on innovative ideas.

He talked them into bringing on more copywriters—especially those with newspaper story experience. Their skills with words far outshone those of the average ad copywriters. He developed catchy slogans and invented product names, including the now-familiar Sunkist, Kleenex, and Kotex. The agency added eye-catching artwork to the advertisements and gave birth to the practice of premiums. Albert's ads encouraged consumers to send in box tops and wrappers, things only those who had purchased the products would be able to procure. In return, they received flatware, cookbooks, and other clever items, endearing the brands to them even more. Every Lord and Thomas client saw their sales go up, and the agency watched its revenues rise.

Albert married Flora Warner in 1902. Two months after their wedding, she contracted typhoid fever. With no antibiotics available at the time, the bacterial infection caused Flora to become incapacitated. She then developed phlebitis and was bedridden for sixteen months from the painful swelling. All the while, Albert was frantic. He was the man who had an answer for nearly any advertising challenge. But he hated being so helpless in the face of his wife's illness, unable to bring the woman he loved back to good health. Fortunately, his business success allowed him to provide her the best medical care money could buy, and Flora survived.[3]

In 1904, Albert was made a one-quarter partner in the agency. Two years later, Ambrose Thomas died, and Albert found himself half owner of the second-largest advertising company in the country. The firm boasted annual billings in excess of $3 million, an unheard-of sum at the time (nearly $85 million today). By 1912, Albert could no longer tolerate his remaining partner's lack of advertising sense, and so he bought him out and became sole owner of Lord and Thomas. With an ample income and a growing family (he and Flora now had three children), the Laskers decided to leave the South Side neighborhood they'd lived in since marrying and looked toward Chicago's increasingly swanky North Shore for a new home. The once-sleepy villages along the Lake Michigan shoreline were becoming popular sites for large estates, built by the city's elite. The Laskers chose Glencoe for their new home, twenty-two miles north of the city. Albert's ulterior motive was Glencoe's Lake Shore Country Club, the leading Jewish club in the area. All the other local clubs barred Jews from joining, and he resolutely refused to set foot in any such club, even as a guest.

During the next decade, Albert expanded the ad firm as well as his investment portfolio. He became a principal owner of the Chicago Cubs, along with William Wrigley, and dipped a toe in political advertising with William

Harding's successful campaign for the presidency. His reward for President Harding's election was being named chairman of the United States Shipping Board. The experience he gained from that appointment gave him a close-up view of how American government functioned. That would serve him well in years to come.

Albert never studied beyond high school, but he greatly valued education, and believed in what it could accomplish. He was also community-minded and philanthropic, like his father. So in January 1928 he and Flora launched the Lasker Foundation for Medical Research at the University of Chicago. They gifted the university a $1 million endowment as seed money for research that would focus on ways to increase the nation's average life span, then just fifty years. The first studies would be on the era's primary killers: hypertension (cardiovascular disease), cancer, and Bright's disease (a type of kidney disease thought to be connected to hypertension). The next year, Albert and his pal Max Epstein, a farsighted businessman and philanthropist, each ponied up $125,000 to build a new university hospital.[4]

A few months later, during the summer of 1929, Albert received a strange telephone call from John Hertz, a friend and Glencoe neighbor. Hertz had not yet begun his car rental business, but he had founded Chicago's Yellow Cab Company and was chairman of a dozen other organizations. The two men had a joint account in the stock market through which both could make changes. "I'm selling everything," Hertz told Albert. The latter was incredulous, because the market was booming. Hertz went on to say he was also selling his personal holdings and that Albert should do the same. Albert was right to trust Hertz's stunning intuition. When the market crashed in October of that year, most of Albert's fortune was preserved. In fact, he was able to make loans to friends and clients alike.[5]

But Albert Lasker had demons. Sometimes he was a highly energetic person: expansive, talkative, outgoing, and extremely creative. Other times he became irritable and an insomniac. Unlike Paul Reinhardt, Albert wasn't an alcoholic; he enjoyed cocktails, however, and all of his characteristics were exacerbated when he drank. He even spent several months at the Henry Phipps Psychiatric Clinic at Johns Hopkins University (where Dr. Adolf Meyer was director). Albert most likely suffered from what is now known as bipolar disorder. It's been discovered that the disorder can run in families, and other Laskers, including his father, Morris, suffered from similar issues.

On top of that, Albert poured every ounce of his being into his business. Family life, friendships, and leisure activities were all sacrificed in his quest to be the best in advertising. He was highly competitive and used every legitimate ploy to win. While the mood swings and Albert's focus on Lord and Thomas must have been difficult for Flora, her love for him never wavered. She supported him, acted as a sounding board, and often encouraged him to go in a direction he might not have considered. Unlike Albert, however, she wasn't terribly interested in the trappings of wealth. Her husband and her children made her wealthy enough.[6]

"All that beauty you see on the screen before you isn't attained without study, improving, perfecting and restyling." And Mary Woodard Reinhardt should know. According to the April 7, 1935, newspaper article that included this opinion, she was an art expert, an editor and—most importantly—a Hollywood fashion authority.[7]

"In the days of the Louis [reigns], the king's mistresses set the fashions and only a few women at court ever saw these style setters," Mary explained. "But, today, you can see the styles for the price of a movie admission fee, and study the science of chic at its source, utilizing the information for your own self improvement."

In the article, Mary opined on the styling of Irene Dunn, Carole Lombard, and Ginger Rogers, all of whom happened to also be featured on her now tremendously popular Hollywood Patterns. The business was going so well, in fact, that Mary had moved into a lovely penthouse on East 52nd Street. This would be just the first home she would occupy in Manhattan's swanky Beekman neighborhood.

The views from her seventeenth-floor windows were spectacular. On one side, the East River glided silently past. On the other, Midtown and the emerging

Rockefeller Center buildings sparkled in the distance. Not only was the pent-house perfect for entertaining, but the two bedrooms and two baths also nicely accommodated Sara, who had moved in with Mary after Frank's death.

And oh, their beautiful terraces! Penthouse gardening was the rage in New York City. If you could afford a penthouse, you could afford help in planning the terrace garden from Bloomingdale's seventh-floor Sky Greenhouse department. Mary had inherited her mother's love of flowers, and the two of them had the terraces planted to such a degree they won numerous prizes. While they didn't have to worry about the neighbors' pets digging up their carefully laid-out beds and artfully placed pots, there was another problem. The gases and soot emitted from the city's chimneys and incinerators choked trees and plants, along with humans. So extreme was the problem that Sara became involved in the Outdoor Cleanliness Association, having brought her nature-loving activism with her from Watertown.

The association, founded in 1931, had as its aim to cleanse the city of litter, filthy streets, and dirty air. Cleaning up New York was, as one reporter called it, "somewhat akin to bathing an elephant."[8] But the association's members (mostly women) were not deterred. Sara went to work persuading the power-generating company Consolidated Edison to put smoke consumers on its stacks, thus reducing the smoke and dirt affecting her rooftop gardens and the lungs of the city's inhabitants. "This was an innovation," Mary remembered, "and of course, Consolidated Edison considered her a terrible, terrible problem, a menace. But she managed this notwithstanding, and she testified against the smoke coming from the industrial and private chimneys in New York, as well as the general lax administration of that smoke."

Mary realized in retrospect that she was much closer to Sara than she had been to her father. Sara taught her daughters to help other people bloom, a lesson Mary never forgot. Both she and Alice were highly influenced by Sara's business acumen and her passion for anything visually beautiful, even though Sara had no formal education in either business or art. The more she thought about it, Mary's own laundry list of interests included fields for which she had had no training, either. She remembered her attentiveness to business and enterprise beginning when she was a child. The selling of goods and services and the development of new products to fulfill human needs intrigued her. Hollywood Patterns was a perfect example, giving women the ability to have lovely new dresses at a low price in the midst of economic struggles.

Her interest in health insurance was born when Mary saw people unable to pay for the medical care they needed. Her hostility to illness—hers or anyone else's—led her to learn more about medical conditions and then try, even if in a very small way, to find money for health investigators (the 1930s term for medical researchers). She was interested in the medical value of psychoanalysis and befriended both Franz Alexander, a physician and psychoanalyst who led a movement exploring the dynamic interrelation between mind and body, and Karl Menninger, a member of the family of psychiatrists who would ultimately found the Menninger Foundation and the Menninger Clinic in Topeka, Kansas.

The common thread among her interests was that Mary Woodard Reinhardt had an overwhelming passion to better the human condition. The frustrating thing was that her income, although comfortable, was nowhere near enough to eradicate all the suffering she knew existed. Why didn't those with means do more? The memory of her experience with the Spanish flu was never far from her mind. When she had enough money, she vowed, she would focus on bettering the health of Americans.

Mary was also becoming very adept in two interconnected realms: engineering fascinating parties and connecting to fascinating people. In an almost chicken-or-egg scenario, it was difficult to tell whether the connecting made for better parties, or vice versa. But it really didn't matter. These two skills would come to serve Mary well in the future. And in the spring of 1939, she was in her element as a hostess.

She had the financial ability to entertain well. In addition to Hollywood Patterns, a second stream of income was flowing from commissions she received from generating business for Paris-born industrial designer Raymond Loewy. After serving in the French army during World War I, Loewy had come to the United States, working as a fashion illustrator until 1929, when he opened his own studio. The press would later call him the Father of Industrial Design, an entirely new industry in the 1930s. Given their joint interests in fashion, art, and design, it was only natural that he and Mary would find themselves in the same circles and that they would hit it off. She was enchanted by his ideas and decided to assist him in finding clients. Whether it was new building facades or commercial interiors, Loewy's work earned him a stellar reputation. And Mary earned a commission on each successful connection she made for him, which brought her annual earnings at the end of the decade to a whopping $25,000 (about half a million dollars today).

She spent her money judiciously, however, collecting tasteful furnishings and, of course, art. This and her reputation as a fabulous hostess brought her to the attention of syndicated columnist Mary Margaret McBride. Under the headline "Noted Decorator Mingles Modern and Antique," McBride explained how Mary kept her terraced penthouse apartment free from the "too-tight decorative feeling," something the writer deplored.

McBride's column—replete with Mary's opinions—elaborated. "'Nothing is more boring than to have furniture all of one country or period,' asserts Mrs. Reinhardt, who several years ago had the first completely modern apartment in the city." The column continued to quote Mary: "'In New York, the consideration of practicality must enter. I wanted mahogany Empire chairs, for instance, upholstered in white, yet in a city as dirty as this, you cannot possibly have white upholstery that does not wash. That meant replacing ancient needlepoint with modern [washable] fabrics.'"

The chairs, along with a Giorgio de Chirico painting of a white horse and a zebra hanging over the mantel and an exquisite harp dating back to 1815, were carefully placed around Mary's paneled living room. McBride's summation: "The furniture [is] a combination of Empire, comfortable modern and ultra-modern mirrored effects. . . . French furniture [sits] cheek by jowl with Italian mirrors and English backgrounds."[9] Against this beautiful tableau, Mary entertained, sometimes joined by Kay Swift or another friend as co-hostess. Typically, a group would meet for dinner at a restaurant and then head to the penthouse for cocktails. The group's size could expand during the warmer months, when Mary would throw open the terrace doors and guests could roam in and out. She described those parties as always extremely interesting events but noted, "People who have done extraordinary things in the world don't always have the best conversation; they have to be stimulated to talk." The beautiful setting and popular gin cocktails (Prohibition had been repealed in 1933) made for great stimulation.

With her entertaining acumen, varied interests, and expanding address book of friends, it was really only a matter of time before the fates put Mary Reinhardt and Albert Lasker in the same place at the same time. On April 1, 1939, Mary was having lunch with her friend Rosita Winston at the 21 Club on West 52nd Street. The seventeen-year-old restaurant had begun life as a speakeasy in Greenwich Village, then moved uptown and soon developed into one of the hottest eateries in Manhattan. It had a very clubby feel about it, as nearly everyone knew everyone else. It was a particularly popular lunch spot among the city's well-knowns.

Seated near the women at a nearby table were two men Mary knew: Lewis Strauss, a wealthy investment banker, and Chicagoan Max Epstein. Mary had met Epstein at the Reinhardt Galleries, where she had impressed her then-husband by selling Epstein a very expensive Frans Hals painting. Another nearby table was occupied by three men. Mary knew two of them: Colonel (later General) "Wild Bill" Donovan, a World War I hero who would go on to greater fame in World War II as head of the Office of Strategic Services, the precursor of the Central Intelligence Agency, and fellow veteran General Robert Wood, who was then president of Sears Roebuck. But the third man, strikingly handsome, was a stranger to Mary.

Donovan knew both Mary and Rosita, and introduced them to the third man, Albert Lasker. Albert, who had been focused on his conversation with his tablemates, smiled weakly at Mary and mumbled an acknowledgment before turning back to the men. When he walked past her a short while later to use the telephone, he didn't even give her a glance. "That man is making a great mistake in not noticing me," Mary thought.

Albert's preoccupation might be explained by a series of recent misfortunes in his personal life. In December 1936, his beloved Flora had died suddenly. Although in ill health throughout their marriage, in the days before her death she looked more radiant and said she was happier than she had ever been. She and Albert were in New York at their luxurious Ritz-Carlton Hotel apartment. Their son, Edward, had just stopped by for a visit. She called out to them from her room, and upon entering they found her unconscious. By the time a doctor arrived, she had died of a cerebral thrombosis.[10]

The grieving widower was nearly inconsolable, racked with guilt at what he might have done to make her life better and to save her from death. To assuage his grief, he threw lavish parties, took a nine-month around-the-world cruise, and tried to figure out what a lonely fifty-six-year-old millionaire was supposed to do with his life. In September 1938, Albert went to California and became the "project" of a friend in the movie industry. Intent on ending Albert's loneliness, the friend hosted nearly nonstop parties. Always on the guest list were glamorous, young, available women, and by the end of the month Albert had met actress Doris Kenyon. In an October 6 gossip piece, Doris denied rumors of a relationship with him. By October 28, the two were sailing for Europe on their honeymoon aboard the luxury liner *Ile de France*.[11]

The honeymoon lasted six weeks, during which time Albert realized his mistake. (Doris probably had, too.) As soon as they had docked in New York City, Albert telephoned his son-in-law Gerhard Foreman, the husband of his elder daughter, Mary, in Chicago. Foreman arrived the next day and took Albert back to Chicago alone, where he lived with the Foremans that winter. A divorce was announced on February 20, 1939, and settlement discussions ensued; they would ultimately take four months.

All of this must have weighed heavily on Albert's mind that day at 21. And even though the three tables finished lunch at the same time, and Lewis Strauss introduced Albert again to Mary, he still didn't exhibit the response to which she was accustomed. On the way down the stairs from the second-floor dining room, Donovan talked Mary up to Albert, praising her enterprising business spirit. When they all arrived in the front hall, Epstein introduced the two a *third* time. Albert snapped out of his stupor then and took a good look at her deep blue eyes, wavy dark hair, and cheeks the color of peonies. As soon as she had left, he began quizzing Donovan about this woman whom everyone seemed to know but him.

Albert wasn't about to let Mary get away. Just months earlier, after the split from Doris, he had declared to a friend, "I'm going to find the right woman if I have to marry *ten* of 'em!"[12] The morning after that first meeting, he telephoned his friend Alva Gimbel, wife of department store mogul Bernard Gimbel. Albert asked her if she knew Mary Reinhardt. Of course she did. Albert had already been invited to spend the following weekend at the Gimbels' country home in Greenwich, Connecticut, and he asked Alva if she might invite Mary to join them. Alva was happy to, but when she called Mary to tell her she wanted her to come for the weekend to meet Albert, Mary demurred. "I have met him," she told her friend in a disinterested-sounding voice. And since her mother was not feeling well, a weekend away was too long. She would, however, come for lunch on Sunday.

Meanwhile, Albert telephoned Max Epstein to hatch another plan. Following instructions, Epstein then called Mary to invite her over for drinks. Mary accidentally dropped the phone at that moment and didn't catch all of the details. Returning to the line, she asked Epstein when. The day after tomorrow at five o'clock, came the answer. Mary agreed. She assumed he was having a large group for a cocktail party at his Ritz-Carlton apartment, so she arrived an hour after the appointed time. When she got there, Albert was the only guest, and he was furious at her tardiness, having an absolute obsession with punctuality. For her part, Mary was confused. According to the conventions of the time, being invited to a five o'clock cocktail party meant she could drop in anytime between five and eight. She hadn't expected there would be only one other guest. And she hadn't expected anyone to be cross with her.

Minutes after blowing his top, however, Albert calmed down, and began a lively conversation with her. They discussed business, gardens, theater, and movies. They discovered many commonalities. He talked of Mill Road Farm, a Chicago estate he'd built a decade earlier. She mentioned she liked boating. He offered her both a tour of the farm and a cruise on his yacht. He talked with such entertaining liveliness that Mary was completely enthralled. He was both factual and amusing, and although he came across as completely self-assured, he was not the least bit pompous.

Lunch at the Gimbels' country home five days later brought another round of conversation between Mary and Albert. On a long walk around the property before they ate, Mary asked him about the situation in Europe and if he thought it would result in war. There was no doubt in Albert's mind that war was exactly what would happen. The time flew by, and the two were so intent on each other, they were an hour late for lunch. When Mary returned home that evening, her mother was alarmed by her daughter's fatigue. "I'm exhausted," Mary explained, "because I've just had lunch with the most exciting man I've ever met!"

But while she found Albert exciting, Mary could also perceive an underlying layer of agitation, nervousness, and distress. And that worried her. As mothers do, Sara was concerned about their age difference. Albert was fifty-eight to Mary's thirty-nine. The nine-year difference between Paul and Mary had been tolerable, but this nearly twenty-year difference was not.

Albert thought Mary resembled a figure in a painting, and he loved that she could hold her own with him in discussions, whether they agreed or not. In Albert, Mary saw all the qualities she admired: good looks, power, business success, creativity, and spontaneity. Despite what she saw as potential trouble beneath the surface, she felt that his eccentricities were not the least bit annoying. In fact, she found them charming. Soon Albert began splitting his time between Chicago and New York.

The divorce from Doris Kenyon became final in June 1939. Although Doris reported that their marriage had been "hasty" and that they had "agreed upon an amicable separation," the Reno, Nevada, decree listed cruelty as her grounds for ending the marriage.[13] Nonetheless, it was a much less stressed Albert who came to New York on June 21 to attend the World's Fair and one of Mary's famous parties. Among the large number of guests she and co-hostess Kay Swift had included was lawyer and utility company head Wendell Willkie, who would be nominated as the Republican presidential candidate the next year. Mary wasn't terribly political, a trait that would soon change. She also considered herself an independent, something else soon to change. But she was attracted to Willkie's personality and thought he would be a good counter to Franklin Roosevelt, who would be running for a third term.

Albert, then a Republican, was, as always, not shy about giving her his opinion. "Well, you may be very intelligent about other things," he told her, "but that's really the craziest idea I've ever heard, to have someone who's the head of a big utility business even discussed as a possible candidate for President. It's just madness."

He shared another opinion with her as well, regarding her long-planned trip to Europe. Mary asked Albert again about the likelihood of war on the Continent, and his opinion hadn't changed. War was coming, he said, and probably by early fall. He told her that if she insisted on going, she had to be home by the middle of July. Hostilities could begin in August, as soon as the harvests were in, he told her. But however persuasive Albert tried to be, Mary never considered staying home.

Her hostess would be British socialite Audrey Pleydell-Bouverie, whose second husband had been Marshall Field III, of Chicago's most famous department store family. She was now married to Peter Pleydell-Bouverie, son of an earl. Bill Donovan had introduced Mary to Audrey, and their shared interests in gardens, art, and beautiful surroundings made the two women immediate friends. Audrey was also allegedly an illegitimate granddaughter of King Edward VII (grandfather to the country's current king), and she moved in high social circles. "Come," she had implored Mary in inviting her to spend time with her in England during the height of the social season, "this may be the end for a long time."

Mary set sail on June 27, and when she arrived at Audrey's London home on July 3 it took her breath away. The 120-year-old mansion in Regent's Park had four and a half acres of gardens and terraces that were only the prologue to its magnificent twenty-six thousand square feet of exquisite rooms. The next day Audrey hosted a formal dinner, and the evening's guests included Adele Astaire (elder sister of Fred), Aly Khan and his first wife (he was the Pakistani prince who would later marry actress Rita Hayworth), and Donovan.

Mary's pal David Sarnoff—the pioneer of radio and television who headed the Radio Corporation of America (RCA)—had given her a letter of introduction to Joe Kennedy, then the U.S. ambassador to Great Britain. The ever-charming Kennedy was as taken with Mary's allure and intelligence as Albert had been. He invited her and the Pleydell-Bouveries to join him and his friends the next night in his box at the Royal Opera House. The group then proceeded to Holland House in Kensington.

This enormous house, situated in the midst of seventy acres, was a scene of social splendor that night. The throngs attending weren't just there for the dancing. King George VI and Queen Elizabeth were present as well. That would be the only ball they attended that season.[14] Mary later remembered, "The queen looked like a beautiful dream, adorned with marvelous jewels. All the women wore tiaras, except me, and the men wore [their military] decorations. It was wonderful.

"Churchill was there," she went on. "I was standing on the stairs with Peter Bouverie, and he introduced me to Mrs. Churchill. Then he turned away and said to me, quietly, 'I can't introduce you to Winston. He's too drunk.'"

The next night was another ball, this one at Blenheim Palace. Sixty miles outside of London, near Oxford, it was the birthplace of Winston Churchill. Mary had visited as a tourist while at Oxford and described it then as dull. But on this night, she found the facade of the palace lighted, along with the gardens, the water terraces, and the lake. She thought it looked like something from a fairy tale. The nine hundred guests dined on the terraces under huge orange tents, scented throughout by six-foot-high incense trees. And as had been the case the night before, the women sparkled in bright gowns and jewels.[15]

But war overshadowed the festivities. Audrey had shared with Mary a powerful premonition she'd had that conflict was just around the corner. She didn't know when, but felt they should enjoy their lives as much as possible in the present. Albert, too, was still concerned. He had sent Mary massive amounts of orchids throughout her stay. But when he sent a telegram imploring her to come back to the United States, she cut her trip short. She made a quick trip to Paris and then boarded the *Ile de France*, leaving the Channel city of Le Havre on July

15. It was the same ship Albert and Doris had been aboard during their honeymoon. Their marital war, however, was nothing compared to what was about to unfold in Europe.

～

Adolf Hitler rose through the ranks of the German government, spewing pan-Germanism, anti-Semitism, and anti-communism with fiery oratory. In what would become the basis for Nazi propaganda, Hitler frequently denounced international capitalism and communism as part of a Jewish conspiracy. When the Great Depression arrived in Europe, it gave Hitler a supreme opportunity. The Nazi Party, he promised, was the way out of the Depression and back to the old German way of life.

Hitler was made dictator of Germany in 1933. And despite the World War I treaty preventing Germany from possessing a military, the new Führer rearmed his country by conscription in 1935. A year later, Germany reoccupied the Rhineland, an area in western Germany near the borders of the Netherlands, Belgium, Luxembourg, and France that had been demilitarized under the Treaty of Versailles. Then, in 1938, Germany annexed Austria, an apparent stepping-stone to expansion.

Next came the two-day orgy of terror known as Kristallnacht, the "Night of Broken Glass." On November 9 and 10, 1938, raging mobs in Germany, Austria, and the Sudetenland freely attacked Jews on the streets, in their homes, and at their places of work and worship. At least ninety-six Jews were killed, hundreds more were injured, and more than a thousand synagogues were burned. Thirty thousand Jews were arrested and sent to concentration camps. Following Kristallnacht, panicky German, Austrian, and Czech Jews flooded into France. Sharing an already limited amount of resources with these immigrants resulted in rabid anti-Semitic feelings throughout the country.

Albert Lasker knew all about anti-Semitism; he had experienced it on a number of occasions during his life. It was one of the things that had driven him to become rich. He was a proud member of the Associated Jewish Philanthropies of Chicago, and felt that only through wealth could he establish standing.

Ironically for Albert and others around the world, the more successful Jews were in business and in life, the more the anti-Semites despised them. Thus Hitler's goal: to see to it they were exterminated completely.

France and Great Britain tolerated Hitler's moves until March 1939, when he seized Bohemia, Moravia, and Slovakia. Allied policymakers abruptly woke up to the fact that Hitler appeared to be marching toward European, if not world, conquest. Indeed he was. At 5:20 a.m. on Friday, September 1, 1939, Adolf Hitler started World War II by dropping German bombs on Poland. The country surrendered on September 27.

But much more was to come, and Audrey's premonitions would prove true. A year later, on September 7, 1940, the German bombing raids on London—the Blitz—began. On the night of September 27, beautiful Holland House was hit by twenty-two incendiary bombs during a ten-hour raid. The mansion was destroyed. Had the attack happened the year before, during that magnificent ball, both monarchs, Winston Churchill, and most of the other British leaders would have been killed, along with Mary Reinhardt.

Chapter 3

—

"You Don't Need
My Kind of Money"

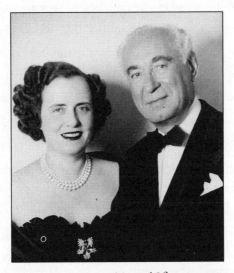

Mary and Albert, circa 1940s.

Three weeks before Hitler began the invasion of Poland, summer was in full swing in the city of Chicago. It's a glorious season in the Windy City, perhaps because it's such a contrast to the harsh winters. But more likely it's the result of the beautiful body of water on which the city sits. Lake Michigan, 118 miles wide, is a magnificent freshwater playground. Municipal beaches fill with bathers, boats bob in the marinas, and baseball discussions abound at lakeside picnics. The weekend of August 11–13, 1939, the Chicago White Sox split a series against the Indians in Cleveland, losing two of three games. But Albert's beloved Cubs were triumphant, sweeping three games from the Pittsburgh Pirates in the friendly confines of Wrigley Field.

Mary had arrived in the city that weekend aboard the 20th Century Limited, the flagship train of the New York Central line. At Grand Central Station, she had walked up the red carpet—rolled out each evening for first-class passengers—and settled into her Pullman. When the train chugged out at 5:30 p.m., she enjoyed cocktails in the observation car, dined cruising through Pennsylvania, and after a comfortable night's rest in her private sleeper, with breakfast served there as well, arrived at Chicago's LaSalle Street Station around 10:00 a.m. A Radcliffe chum, Janet Fairbank, was there to meet her.

Janet was building a career as a professional soprano, and would be singing later in the month at Chicago's Grant Park. But this weekend was to be one of landscape tours. Both women loved driving through the luxurious northern suburbs along the Lake Michigan shoreline, viewing the beautiful estates and gardens. Mary had an additional destination for their itinerary this summer, however: Sunday lunch at Albert's Mill Road Farm. Mary saw at once that his description of it the previous year at Max Epstein's apartment hadn't done it justice. She would later say, "It was incomparably the best place in the Middlewest and probably the best-run and best all over country house in the United States."

The property was located in Lake Forest, about twenty-four miles north of the city. Albert had bought the 480 acres in 1921 from meatpacking king Louis Swift, paying $1,000 an acre. As it had been with his earlier Glencoe purchase twelve miles south, part of his motivation for the expansive property was that Jews were still banned from membership at any of the exclusive area country clubs. So Albert decided to create his own country club. And when it was all completed, his Mill Road Farm came in at a price tag of $3.5 million (over $56 million today).[1]

After traveling the curving, tree-lined drive, visitors arrived at the twenty-five-thousand-square-foot residence, built in the French Provincial style. The mansion had fifty-six rooms, including suites for Albert, his wife, Flora (who was still alive at the time the house was built), and each of their three children. Each suite had a private bath. Half a dozen guest rooms, four sitting rooms, a wine cellar, a pressing room, a silver room, and a dozen servants' rooms were also part of the main building. Flora had overseen all of the decorating and garden planning. The Laskers enjoyed entertaining, and the guests poured in.

Scattered around the manicured grounds were twenty-five ancillary buildings, including greenhouses, a twelve-car garage, a guesthouse to accommodate eight overnight visitors, and a superintendent's residence. For leisure activity, there were two tennis courts and a 100-by-40-foot swimming pool, complete with two large bathhouses. There was a barn for the herd of prize Guernsey cattle, a stable, and chicken houses.

And then there was Albert's pride and joy: the $1 million eighteen-hole golf course. It was one of the few private courses in America at the time, and after playing it, famed professional golfer Bobby Jones proclaimed it among the top three courses in the country. It was beautiful to look at, and tough, with a par of 70. Being invited to play at Albert's course was a big deal. His friend John Hertz attested, "There isn't anybody in Chicago who doesn't want to play his course. . . . There just isn't a place to compare with it."

Despite the fact that the estate required a staff of more than fifty—making Lasker the largest employer in the Lake Forest area at the time—Albert was as interested in comfort as in grandeur. His was more of a welcoming country house than an over-the-top replica of a royal palace. Mary had that impression, too. "It was in very beautiful taste, it had marvelous gardens . . . and all quite unpretentious-looking at the same time, not at all grand-looking. . . . It also had a small movie house, which I thought was enchanting."

After a tour of the house, Mary, Janet, Albert, his son, Edward, and several other guests enjoyed a wonderful lunch on the terrace that sunny Sunday afternoon. Leaving Chicago on Monday, Mary went on to San Francisco to attend the Golden Gate International Exposition. While she was there, Albert telephoned her, saying he was worn out. Although he didn't articulate it at the time, there were a number of possible reasons for his fatigue. He had recently been involved in a trial, not as a major player, but he had been called upon to explain his relationship, and that of Lord and Thomas, with the defendant. In addition, he was growing weary of the pressures of the advertising business. But probably most concerning of all to Albert was his conflicted feelings over his relationship with Mary. She intrigued him. She enthralled him. And she terrified him. He was gun-shy after the debacle of his second marriage.

Friends on both sides were watching the couple as well, concerned about a possible explosion, as both Mary and Albert were extremely headstrong. But some years later, one of those friends admitted his error: "They both had character and intelligence, and above all, love, that simple and scarce thing. You couldn't be around them and not know it."[2]

But on the telephone that day, Albert told Mary that a friend had sent a private plane with a nurse for him, and that he was headed to a ranch in Tucson to rest. He stayed for more than two months, in near-complete isolation. Once a week he was driven to the nearest phone, ninety miles away, to call Mary. A doctor in Arizona suggested that he had an adrenal gland malfunction, which somewhat mollified Albert; at least he wasn't mentally ill, as he had feared. But Mary wasn't satisfied with the diagnosis. When he came to New York in November, she convinced Albert to see a world-renowned internist, who in turn referred him to renowned endocrinologists. All tests came back negative; they could find nothing physically wrong with him.

Mary actually suspected his issues were more of an emotional nature, and she gradually began selling him on the idea of psychoanalysis. Albert went somewhat begrudgingly. But before long, he was fascinated by the process, and he saw the psychiatrist four or five times a week. It wasn't formal psychoanalysis, and he didn't lie down on a couch. Rather, doctor and patient talked, man to man. They discussed Albert's dreams, his father's domination, and his distress at feeling as though he had been a public success but a private failure. The analysis did him a great deal of good, so much so that he later told a friend, "You know what it did for me? It taught me to forgive myself."[3]

That realization was monumental. And it was followed by an urge to begin divesting himself of things that connected him to the past. The first to go was Mill Road Farm, which he donated to the University of Chicago in December 1939. Shocking as that may seem, Albert concluded that the estate was very much an emblem of the Roaring Twenties, now a bygone era. He was a trustee of the university, and he hoped it would be of some use to them. If, after two years, they hadn't figured out what to do with it, they were free to dispose of it. This they did, selling it off in pieces. But not before Albert rented it back from them the next two summers. And he wouldn't be there alone.

〜

By 1940, understanding of hypertension (high blood pressure) and diseases of the brain had not progressed much since the turn of the century. Some doctors even espoused that high blood pressure was good for the body. In 1931, cardiologist John Hay opined, "The greatest danger to a man with high blood pressure lies in its discovery, because then some fool is certain to try and reduce it."[4]

Others suggested that cerebral hemorrhages, the brain bleeds that often result from high blood pressure, were self-inflicted, as expressed in a 1939 newspaper article: "It remains a fact, that most of those who die of cerebral hemorrhage have contributed toward the fatality." The writer felt they occurred because of "high-gear living, over-eating and drinking, over exertion, and poorly regulated routine of exercise and rest." They might also be the "result of rapidly eating, accompanied by heated discussion."[5]

No wonder that cerebral hemorrhages ranked among the top five killers in the United States. And there were very few treatment options. Most patients were given phenobarbital (to slow the activity of their brain and nervous system), advised to follow a low-fat, low-sodium diet and get plenty of rest. With so little useful information, it's not difficult to imagine Mary's despair when her mother died suddenly of a cerebral hemorrhage on January 9, 1940. Mary and Alice took her body back to Watertown for a funeral at the Congregational Church and burial in the city's Oak Hill Cemetery next to Frank. Tragically, Mary had now lost both parents to the same disease. But her emotions went beyond grief. "I was deeply resentful that nothing could be done to help her. It was considered something like the will of God, that one couldn't do anything about it medically, and this I bitterly resented."

Unlike at the time of Frank's death, however, Mary now had Albert in her life. His experience of Flora's sudden death gave him a true understanding of her grief. They soon began seeing each other very frequently in New York, being invited to parties as a couple. One of those events introduced them to Anna Rosenberg. They all had a great deal in common. Aside from Albert and Anna both being Jewish, he was impressed with her publicity acumen. Mary thoroughly identified with her drive, networking skills, and never-say-no attitude (something Mary would also soon be known for).

Like Mary, Anna was unique in that she was ahead of her time. And when she spoke, people listened. There were two reasons for this. The most visible reason was her attention-grabbing hats, and she admitted to having a weakness for silly ones. When she first entered the political scene, her friends asked her not to wear any of her "unconservative" hats. She disregarded their advice and wore exactly what she pleased, and, as a result, she was much happier. The second, more substantive reason people listened was her extensive expertise in labor relations, an unusual specialty for women in that era.

Born in Hungary in 1901, she came to the United States with her family eleven years later. As a young adult, she made a speech about the women's suffrage movement, which brought her to the attention of a New York political organizer. That, in turn, led her to open Anna Rosenberg Associates, a public relations firm she would maintain until her death. Her reputation and client list grew, as she managed campaigns for New York aldermen, congressmen, and Mayor Fiorello La Guardia.

When Franklin Roosevelt was elected governor of New York in 1929, it was Anna he frequently consulted on labor matters. That relationship would serve her well. She became a regional director of his National Recovery Administration in 1936, and the next year was given the same title with the Social Security Board, where her job was to interpret and implement the terms of the Social Security Act. In every case, Anna shattered glass ceilings. Very often she was the only woman at the table, be it the dining table or the negotiating table. "Too often people change their personalities, especially women," she later said. "They try to compete with men on men's terms, which is silly. They should compete on their own terms."[6]

Although they were the same age, Mary learned a great deal from Anna. They dined together, went to the theater together, and even vacationed together. One day at lunch, Anna confided to Mary and Albert that she was ill and would be leaving that afternoon for the Mayo Clinic. She planned to travel aboard the 20th Century Limited to Chicago and then on to the clinic in Rochester, Minnesota, nearly four hundred miles to the north. Albert—always a man to lend a hand to someone he thought highly of—felt an over-the-top urge to help her, even though this independent woman never indicated any need whatsoever.

When Anna descended the train's steps in Chicago the next morning, therefore, she was stunned to find an attendant with a wheelchair and the city's commissioner of health waiting for her. This was the culmination of Albert's elaborate work. The men physically picked Anna up, put her in the chair, and wheeled her off. Her frantic protests went unheard; they calmly explained that these had been Mr. Lasker's orders. She was taken to the commissioner's home, where she was put to bed until her train to Rochester left that evening. At the end of it all, her health issue resolved itself nicely, and the friendship was even more firmly cemented.[7]

Mary became Mrs. Albert Lasker on June 21, 1940. She and Albert had agreed that if they started issuing invitations to their wedding, they'd wind up having to invite several hundred for fear of insulting those not included. That was far too much hoopla, so they didn't invite anyone. For a wedding between a successful businesswoman and an incredibly rich adman, the City Hall ceremony was remarkably minimal. It was presided over by New York Supreme Court justice Lloyd Church, and the judge's two bedraggled-looking clerks were the witnesses. When it was over, Judge Church said, "I believe this is all that's required under the laws of the state of New York. Two dollars, please." And that was that.

As if their wedding ceremony hadn't been quirky enough, the honeymoon was quirkier still. It began on a small yacht Albert had chartered for a two-day cruise on Long Island Sound. Next, they traveled to Philadelphia, checking into the luxurious Barclay Hotel, to attend the Republican presidential convention, taking place June 24–28. Without the convenience of today's vast media options and pre-election debates, the conventions of this era involved a great deal of drama. Candidates had to rely on the strength of their floor delegates to earn a nomination. Albert, still a loyal Republican, served as a delegate from Illinois. He helped swing the state's delegates to Wendell Willkie, which in turn put Willkie over the top and put him on the ballot. Mary had never attended a political convention, so to have her first experience include the nomination of the man she supported was exciting.

The newlyweds returned to New York for a week, and then continued the convention-themed honeymoon by heading to Chicago on July 13 for the Democratic convention. Anna was already there, thrilled to welcome and congratulate them. Her boss and friend, Franklin Roosevelt, was trying for an unprecedented third nomination. Albert had met FDR in 1937, when an out-of-the-blue lunch invitation arrived from the White House. The Republican adman and the Democratic president had an amicable lunch, during which the president dominated the conversation. (Albert's biographer, John Gunther, suggested that perhaps FDR wanted to discuss American isolationism should war come to Europe. But that conversation never materialized.) Now, three years later, Roosevelt was successful in his renomination.

When it was over, the Laskers took to the water once again, this time to cruise Lake Michigan aboard Albert's yacht, the *Kenkora II*, built in 1930 for $150,000 ($2.5 million in today's money). Albert co-owned the ship with Kenneth Smith, whose father had founded Pepsodent toothpaste, which became one of Lord and Thomas's biggest clients. When Pepsodent had financial troubles during the market crash and ensuing Depression, Albert loaned them $100,000 to keep it afloat. The *Kenkora II* figured in as part of his repayment.

The coal-black ship was described as "one of the most modern yachts on the Great Lakes." Nearly two hundred feet in length, it had a crew of two dozen. And on board, it was hard to remember that it was a ship and not a luxurious private home. The twenty-by-thirty-foot living room boasted a grand piano, while one of the wood-paneled walls of the "tap room"—a combination bar and smoking room—featured an inlaid panel depicting the skyline of Chicago. On the lower deck and running the entire width of the yacht was the enormous owner's stateroom, along with five guest rooms, each with a private bath. Happily for Mary, the rooms were air-conditioned; she detested heat.

The plan was to cruise up the shoreline, but due to rough waters, they only got as far as Milwaukee. They stayed three days, traveling to nearby Oconomowoc to visit the Pabsts. Mary's school chum Pauline Pabst had married Raimund Wurlitzer (of organ fame) two decades earlier, with Mary as a bridesmaid. True to Pabst fashion, the visit was lively and great fun. The Laskers were hoping to then cross the lake to visit Michigan friends, but the water remained rough. So they went instead to Mill Road Farm, which Albert had rented back from the university for the summer, and stayed until early September. Back in New York, they moved into a temporary apartment on the southern edge of Central Park.

No matter how much she loved Albert, Mary wasn't about to become a kept woman. (She had never gotten over her father's parsimony.) She asked Albert what kind of budget they should live on. He found that amusing and told her it didn't matter. "I don't want to be mixed up with your money," she informed him. "You live on yours, and I'll live on mine." He was astounded but agreed, though he offered to at least cover the rent and grocery bills, while she could pay for her clothing and her large telephone bills. That didn't mollify her.

"I don't want to be taken over," she insisted. "I want to be able to spend what's mine any way I like." He was still unsure, but respected her independence. Not long after, a woman visited Mary seeking a considerable donation for her charity. Mary explained that while she'd like to donate, she couldn't afford that sum. The woman looked around the beautifully decorated apartment and went away unconvinced. Mary thought the story was amusing and shared it that evening with Albert's son, who was not amused. He went straight to his father, telling him it was scandalous that Mary didn't have a large amount of capital in the bank.

The next day, Albert asked Mary to come to his office. He presented her with a check for a million dollars. "There are no strings on this at all," he explained. "Invest it at your will. It embarrasses me to think you have no substantial funds of your own." Just as he had respected her independence, Mary respected his generosity and kind heart. She took the check and immediately invested it in blue chip stocks. There was no more discussion of whose dollars belonged to whom.[8]

⚊

In 1939, before Mary met Albert, she had gone to a meeting of the newly formed Birth Control Federation of America, founded by Margaret Sanger. In no time, Mary came to admire both the cause and the woman. Margaret's mother had conceived eighteen times and birthed eleven live babies before she died at the age of forty-nine. Margaret was the sixth of the eleven children, and she spent her youth doing household chores and caring for her younger siblings. As an adult she had worked in hospitals in the poor sections of New York, where, on more than one occasion, she was called to the home of a woman who had attempted self-induced abortion and was bleeding to death.

At the time, the words "birth control" were illegal to say out loud or put into print. Contraception was available (in the form of condoms), but only if you knew where to look and had the means to pay. That meant that for women in poorer communities, whose finances were already stretched to the max, it was not accessible. Margaret became their champion, her outspokenness on the topic landing her in headlines and jail cells.

After they married, Mary told Albert she wanted to raise money for the organization to help educate women on pregnancy prevention. She was shocked when Albert told her that he, too, knew Margaret Sanger and had donated to another organization she had previously been associated with. The Laskers scheduled a meeting with Margaret. Mary gave her $10,000; Albert gave her a lesson in advertising. He boldly suggested she change the organization's name. The term "birth control," he felt, was too negative. He suggested calling the organization Planned Parenthood. The organization's leadership agreed.[9]

That led Albert to later ask his wife, "What do you want to get done in life? What are you most interested in?"

"Well," Mary replied, with little hesitation, "I'm really most interested in trying to get legislation for national health insurance. I'm interested in cancer research and research against tuberculosis." She summed it up by telling him she just wanted to alleviate suffering.

Enthusiastic as always, Albert replied, "Well, for that you don't need my kind of money. You need federal money, and I will show you how to get it." His tenure as head of the Shipping Board, one of the largest federal agencies in the country at that time, had taught him a great deal about legislation and the psychology of politicians. It was all about connections, he told her. So Mary asked Anna for a letter of introduction to First Lady Eleanor Roosevelt, who was also interested in birth control. In response, Mrs. Roosevelt invited Mary to come to the White House for dinner on October 14, 1941, and to plan to spend the night.

Mary arrived in the afternoon, went to a meeting Mrs. Roosevelt had organized with the surgeon general, and then met the First Lady for tea. An hour later, she was escorted to a second-floor guest room. When she was ready to go down to dinner, she found President Roosevelt sitting in his wheelchair and waiting for her outside the elevator. They chatted as they descended to the Red Room, where the president made cocktails for the two of them. He did the same for fellow guests Anna Rosenberg and Fiorello La Guardia, as well as for Mrs. Roosevelt when she came in.

The dinner conversation meandered. FDR shared the news that he'd spoken with Secretary of State Cordell Hull, who thought the outlook for both Japan and Russia was not good. Lightening up, the president changed the topic to gossip about Hollywood stories, until Mrs. Roosevelt mentioned that Mary had had some success that afternoon discussing birth control with the surgeon general. FDR dismissed the topic, saying it was a political hot potato, and the conversation then drifted to sports.

Despite meeting the next day with the secretary of labor, Frances Perkins, under whose purview the Children's Bureau fell, Mary's trip failed in getting the attention for the birth control education program she had hoped for. Its name was problematic (as Albert had noted), the politically powerful Catholic Church was against it, and the subject was so taboo they couldn't garner newspaper or

radio attention. Probably saddest of all, it just wasn't a topic Washington politicians (primarily wealthy white men) were interested in. Thinking of the horrific
stories Margaret Sanger had told her, Mary felt defeated by the public's lethargy
and its ignorance of—and embarrassment at—the topic.

Mrs. Roosevelt invited her to come back to the White House on December
8. They would have a luncheon for anyone Mary wanted to invite, including
those from the Public Health Service (PHS). Along with their representatives,
individuals from the Birth Control Federation were invited as well. And then
the unthinkable happened.

On December 7, the Imperial Japanese Navy launched unprovoked attacks
on seven Pacific targets: Pearl Harbor in Hawaii, Guam, Wake Island, Midway
Island, Malaya, Hong Kong, and the Philippines. Shortly after noon on December 8, just as the luncheon was beginning, FDR left the White House to address
a joint session of Congress. Mrs. Roosevelt and their thirty-four-year-old son
James accompanied him in the presidential motorcade. At 12:29 p.m., Roosevelt
began to speak: "Yesterday, December 7, 1941, a date which will live in infamy,
the United States of America was suddenly and deliberately attacked by naval
and air forces of the Empire of Japan. . . . I ask that the Congress declare . . . a
state of war."[10]

Mary served as the luncheon hostess until Mrs. Roosevelt returned from
the Capitol. But everyone was in such a state of agitation, there wasn't much
enthusiasm to discuss anything, and Mary returned home, again disappointed.
But as Albert pointed out to her, thanks to her relationship with Anna, she had
now met both the president and the First Lady, along with a variety of others in
government. In retrospect, she would remember that this was her first foray into
working toward better public health. And over the coming months and years,
her friendship with Mrs. Roosevelt, whom she greatly admired, blossomed.

As 1941 and then 1942 passed, the war consumed everyone's thoughts, regardless of social or economic status. In the spring of 1943, Mary read the recently

released *Victory Through Air Power*, written by Russian American pilot Major Alexander de Seversky. De Seversky wrote that the current American military emphasis was on building tanks, while the priority for building aircraft was very low. In addition to increasing aircraft production, de Seversky also advocated for planes that could carry large bomb loads and have great range and speed. America had nothing comparable to the English Spitfires or Hurricanes that had saved Great Britain during the Blitz of 1940–1941.

If what he said was true, Mary could see that America, and by extension the Allied forces, were in great peril of defeat. She told Albert her concerns and encouraged him to read the book. He replied that her suggestion that the United States had inadequate defense planning couldn't possibly be right; she had to be mistaken. A knock-down, drag-out discussion ensued. "All I ask you to do," she said, summoning as much influence as she could muster, "is read the book." His love for her won out. "All right, I'll read the book." He was sure she was crazy, but by the time he got to the last page, he, too, was convinced, and shocked beyond words.

Albert wanted to meet Major de Seversky, who was speaking in New York a few weeks later. So Mary went. Afterward, she approached him, introducing herself and inviting him to their home to meet Albert. De Seversky surprised her by saying he already knew him, a fact Albert had apparently forgotten. When they met again, de Seversky reemphasized his beliefs, and Albert promised that he and Mary would help get the pilot-turned-author's message into the right hands. After all, money and position have their privileges.

They started by scheduling a meeting with Frank Knox, secretary of the navy. The secretary listened politely and invited them on two cruises down the Potomac on his houseboat. But he was not moved by the Laskers' passion for airpower. Albert next used his advertising contacts, first persuading NBC to grant de Seversky considerable time on the radio, and then securing print coverage for him with Scripps-owned newspapers. Intent on bringing pressure to the people in charge of war production, and to help them better understand the importance of airpower, the Laskers also purchased two thousand autographed copies of *Victory Through Air Power*. Along with a personal letter, they sent them to members of Congress, members of the cabinet, and major opinion-makers in the country, including Walt Disney.

Disney was no stranger to war involvement. Immediately after the 1941 Japanese attack, the Disney studios had been converted into a government information machine that helped the American public understand the war's progress. Now Disney saw the immense value in de Seversky's message. Following discussions with the major and the Laskers, the studio made a movie (also called *Victory Through Air Power*) based on the facts in the book. Albert served as a consultant.

Four days before the movie's July 17, 1943, release, the Laskers threw a huge dinner party at the Waldorf-Astoria. One thousand guests were treated to a private screening. De Seversky invited the influential people he knew, and the Laskers did the same. The major's media exposure grew, yet his friends in the Army Air Corps were cautious about espousing his ideas to politicians or the president, a profoundly navy-minded man. It was only after the Laskers' final step, getting a copy of the film to British prime minister Winston Churchill (it was already being shown in British theaters and receiving rave reviews), that it was shown to FDR when he and Churchill attended the first Quebec Conference in 1943. Roosevelt was mightily impressed, grasping and embracing the concept of air superiority.[11]

The *Victory Through Air Power* project may seem far afield from Mary's passion to improve the health of Americans. But some version of war would weave its way in and out of her life for a long time to come.

—

One of the Laskers' destinations to escape New York's cold winter temperatures was the Sunshine State. Albert had first visited Florida in 1925. He fell so in love with it, he bought 100 feet of Atlantic Ocean frontage on Collier Avenue in Miami. Costing $175,000 ($3 million in today's money, but probably worth double that given the location), the mansion he built was designed by the same architect who had envisioned his Mill Road Farm. Albert's gregarious personality brought him into the social sphere of full-time Miami residents Dan and

Florence Mahoney. And it wasn't long after Albert met Mary that she, too, became friends with the Mahoneys.

Florence liked Mary immediately. "I liked anybody who was intelligent," she proclaimed, and Mary was very intelligent. But it was their shared interest in health topics that became their bond. From birth control to mental hygiene, cancer, and beyond, they were never at a loss for conversation. "We didn't think of backing any 'causes' at all," Florence later explained, "we were just talking about things we were interested in."[12]

But the Mahoneys were certainly connected. Dan's first wife (who had died in 1921) was the daughter of James Cox, a man who'd been a congressman and a three-term Ohio governor and taken a run at the presidency. He was also the founder of the News League, a large newspaper company (that, as Cox Enterprises, has many more divisions now). Cox had hired Mahoney in 1919, and when Dan became company vice president charged with overseeing the development of the company's *Miami Daily News,* the Mahoneys moved to Florida.

The Laskers had sold their Miami estate in 1942; now their winter sojourns were spent at the luxurious Whitehall in Palm Beach. The palatial estate had once been the home of Florida railroad magnate and Standard Oil co-founder Henry Flagler. After he and his wife died, the property became a swank hotel. The mansion's majestic first-floor rooms were the hotel's public areas. And while a twelve-story tower of guest rooms had been built, the Laskers always secured one of the fifteen original second-story bedroom suites, reserved exclusively for the high-end crowd.

When they arrived on the first day of March in 1944, Mary dove into a book she had brought along, hardly light reading for lounging in the hotel's coconut grove. *Science at War,* written by George W. Gray, had been published the previous December. Gray wrote in the preface that if "a humane world society is to be the fruit of our victory [speaking of the then ongoing world war], organized science will be as necessary to the waging of peace as it has been to the waging of war."[13] Mary was intrigued.

Medical research, Gray continued, was being done by the Office of Scientific Research and Development (OSRD)'s Committee on Medical Research (CMR).

The presidentially mandated OSRD, created in July 1941, answered directly to FDR and had carte blanche to fast-track scientific research to support the war effort. The CMR, which was packed with medical heavyweights, was aiming to develop much-needed new drugs, particularly for the troops fighting in the Pacific Theater. Much was done in secrecy, completely under the radar of the public (it was OSRD that was responsible for the Manhattan Project). But the CMR's work was less locked down, and ultimately successful in a number of breakthroughs: penicillin for infections, sulfa drugs for treating wounds and burns, cortisone, a synthetic form of quinine (to cure malaria), and others. More importantly, Mary realized that a great deal of money was flowing from the government for medical research. In fact, by the end of the war, there had never been so much federal spending heading into that pot.

Why, then, couldn't—or wouldn't—the government do the same thing in peacetime, as Gray suggested? When the Lakers trekked down to Miami at the end of the month to spend their annual several weeks with the Mahoneys, Mary was keen to share all of this with Florence, whose experience in the newspaper world made her very comfortable setting meetings with politicians. "She didn't see any problem going to see a governor in a state house about health issues," Mary explained, "or going to see people in Washington, for that matter."

After hearing what Mary had read in *Science at War,* Florence encouraged her to look into it further when she got back to New York. "I'm always puzzled because the human race is full of illness and medical problems," Mary told her. "Why hasn't there been more of an effort to find out how to control major diseases, and more dynamic attempts to raise funds?"

It puzzled Florence as well, and Mary continued, "The problems are so enormous and have to be attacked on such a large scale in order to get anything done in any relatively short space of time. There's no reason why federal money shouldn't be used. [It's] only our money in another pocket."

Indeed it is.

Chapter 4

"We Were the Grassroots Rising"

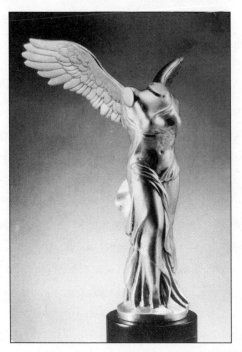

*The Albert Lasker Award, inspired by
the Winged Victory of Samothrace.*

"Colonel W. C. Menninger Wins First Lasker Award." The small
article following this minor headline on November 9, 1944,
was only a preview of what the newly created Lasker Awards
would become.[1] The awards were born as the result of two occurrences.

The first was the day in late 1942 when Albert came home from a lunch
and declared, "Mary, I have decided to give up Lord and Thomas." Mary was
shocked at such a drastic move and suggested he think it over for forty-eight

hours. He did; his decision remained unchanged, as did his reasons. First, he was tired. He had been associated with the company for forty-four years, beginning at a weekly salary of $10. Now the company was worth tens of millions, yet none of his children was interested in taking over. Second, Albert was bored. The ad business he had known, loved, and created was changing, and he wasn't interested in retraining himself. Third, most of his wealth was tied up in Lord and Thomas's cash reserves. Cashing out would give him more money than he could spend and satisfy his last reason: Albert had always been philanthropic; Mary had now ignited in him an even greater interest.

But selling straight out wasn't an option; there couldn't be a Lord and Thomas without Albert. So he engineered a liquidation of the existing firm, with plans for the company's three senior partners to create a new incarnation of the firm in its stead. He had sounded out each of the agency's chief clients (including Sunkist, Kimberly-Clark, Armour Meats, Pepsodent, Lucky Strike, and Lockheed) to ensure they would stay with the new firm. Meanwhile, the three executives—Emerson Foote, holding down the New York office; Fairfax Cone, in Chicago; and Don Belding, on the West Coast—ponied up a minor sum for the company's furniture and other assets. And on January 1, 1943, the new Foote, Cone and Belding debuted. These three men, who had never worked in the same room before, now owned an agency that had done three-quarters of a billion dollars in business over the past seventy years. Albert never interfered in anything they did subsequently, but he remained available for consultation if they needed him. Happily, Emerson Foote remained a friend for life.[2]

Albert was later asked if he missed it. "The Lasker of the advertising business died in 1942," he replied. "I never think of him, and I'm not sure I ever knew the man."[3]

This momentous step led to the second occurrence that resulted in the Lasker Awards. The foundation that Albert and Flora had created at the University of Chicago in 1928 (and their $1 million endowment) had not produced the research bounty they had hoped for. Albert had been busy with the agency, and it was difficult to maintain dedicated people to keep an eye on how the research was progressing. Eventually he agreed to release the money for general university purposes. When Mary had heard this story early on in their marriage, she was distraught at the lost opportunity. So the Laskers began a discussion about a new foundation.

Albert was interested in helping what he called philanthropic "bargains": organizations, people, and causes that didn't get much attention from larger institutions. The federal government was spending nearly nothing on medical investigations; virtually all research money came from universities and private foundations. The era's preeminent grant-making body was the Rockefeller Institute for Medical Research, founded by John D. Rockefeller, who had endowed it with $65 million (more than $1 billion in today's money). The institute was located less than a mile from the Laskers' Beekman Place town house, so they went to visit Dr. Alan Gregg, the institute's director of medical sciences, for advice on how they might help in current research. Since cancer was such an interest to them, they asked what was being done in that area. "Nothing," Dr. Gregg replied, explaining that—despite the institute's enormous financial pool—they were only spending about $50,000 on cancer research annually. Mary asked why so little had been allocated. "Because there aren't any ideas," Dr. Gregg answered.

They went home and pondered this, and Mary told Albert that if there weren't any ideas, they should help create some. "If you have money, and if people are employed to work in an area," she reasoned, "eventually they will generate ideas." So with a $50,000 investment from their personal funds, they created the Albert and Mary Lasker Foundation in December 1942. Interest from the initial amount would help them achieve their mission of promoting "health through education and research."

A year and a half later, as Mary was making out her will, she was musing aloud with her attorney about her desire to leave her money in the form of awards for researchers. She was suddenly struck by an idea. Why not do it while she and Albert were still alive to enjoy it? And then she had another idea.

"Darling, [y]our birthday is a great problem," Mary wrote to her husband on April 30, 1944. "I would like to make you a present that would bring you some particular joy or honor. Joy, I can't produce in new ways so I will have to go on to honor.

"This is to certify that when we have found a suitable agency for presenting the prizes, I personally wish to see an annual prize for medical research for the cure of cancer to be called the Albert Lasker Prize for Cancer Research. And I hope the person who discovers the cure will receive it within ten years. Love to you, my angel."

The initial amount of the Lasker Prize was a modest $1,000, but the organization they selected to make the presentation of the inaugural award was the perfect choice: the late Clifford Beers's National Committee for Mental Hygiene, of which Mary had been made secretary just two months earlier. It gave her great pleasure to recognize Dr. William C. Menninger for his "outstanding service in mental hygiene." With more attention being given to medical research, surely the award for a cancer cure would not be far off.

Sixteen years earlier, in 1928, Senator Matthew Neely, a West Virginia Democrat, stood before his Senate colleagues, addressing them with his soon-to-be-legendary eloquence and drama.

"I propose," he began, "to speak of a monster that is more insatiable than the guillotine; more destructive to life and health and happiness than the World War . . . more terrifying than any other scourge that has ever threatened the existence of the human race. . . . The name of this loathsome, deadly and insatiate monster is cancer."

Neely wanted the Senate to take a serious stand against the disease, and to provide the funding needed to cure it. "Medical science," he continued, "has conquered yellow fever, diphtheria, typhoid and smallpox. . . . But in spite of all that physicians, surgeons, chemists, biologists, and all other scientists have done, cancer remains unconquered."[4]

The Senate passed Neely's bill to fund cancer research, but despite his pleas and his declaration that cancer was "costing the United States almost $800 million a year," the bill did not pass in the House. Eight years later, fellow Democrat Maury Maverick of Texas took up the charge by introducing a bill to establish a national cancer institute. Maverick met with President Roosevelt to discuss his cancer research effort. FDR suggested the easiest way to get Congress on board was to tack an amendment about cancer to the appropriation for the current hot topic in health: venereal disease.

Another bill similar to Maverick's, meanwhile, was also making the rounds, sponsored by Washington Democrat Homer Bone. All of Bone's Senate colleagues were on board except for one. That senator's position was that government interference in cancer research was a step closer to socialized medicine, something Mary would hear often in the future. Not long after, however, the senator's wife was diagnosed with cancer. He became desperate to find her a cure, and withdrew his previous opposition to the bill. Bone also enlisted freshman representative Warren Magnuson to introduce a twin bill in the House. With the energy of Bone, Magnuson, and Neely behind cancer research, along with support from Maverick, joint hearings took place in both houses of Congress in July 1937. A compromise bill was enacted on July 23, and the National Cancer Institute Act was signed by President Roosevelt two weeks later.[5]

The National Cancer Institute (NCI) became the federal government's primary agency to investigate the cause, diagnosis, and treatment of cancer. Money in the act provided for a state-of-the-art laboratory space, and Senator Bone himself broke ground for the new building on October 3, 1938. However, when the shadow of war in Europe became the real thing and America went on high alert to protect itself, research took a back seat. The "scourge," however, kept killing.

⟶

Mary had first become aware of cancer when she was five. One day her mother took her to visit Mrs. Belter, their laundress in Watertown, who had recently undergone a double mastectomy. On the way, Sara explained that to save Mrs. Belter's life, her breasts had been removed. Mary was incredulous: "What do you mean? Cut off?" Sara confirmed it. When they arrived, Mrs. Belter was lying on a low bed in a small, shabby room, her seven children crowded around her. Mary never forgot the miserable sight. Even then it made her furious. Why could no one help this poor woman?

Cancer's next target in Mary's realm was her good friend Kay Swift's mother, Ellen Dorr, who had died of breast cancer in 1928. That, too, had made Mary furious. But she also saw that no one seemed the least bit hurried to learn more about the disease. To Mary's mind, that was not just confounding but inhumane.

Fourteen years later, after the Laskers' conversation about cancer research with Dr. Gregg, Mary began a collection of clippings and pamphlets, including a brochure from the American Society for the Control of Cancer (ASCC), head-quartered in New York's Empire State Building.

When Florence Mahoney came to New York for a visit in the fall of 1943, she and Mary paid the society a call; Mary thought perhaps the Lasker Foundation could help further their research. Given that so much time had passed since Mrs. Dorr's death, surely they must have many projects in the works. But Mary would be disappointed. When she asked Dr. Clarence Little, then the managing director, how much of the $350,000 they had raised that year went to research, he told them that none of it had. They asked why, but no real answer was forth-coming, which prompted Mary to later sniff, "They weren't going to eliminate cancer, they were just going to control it."

Mary knew that all of the society's fundraising efforts rested on the shoul-ders of the Women's Field Army, a volunteer group that was a branch of the ASCC. The nationwide group of thirty thousand had been organized around 1936 to go door-to-door to educate women about cancer symptoms and preven-tion, because "family health is the woman's job."[6] Well-intentioned as the Field Army was, they were more or less led by the society's board of directors—all doctors, all men, and primarily all New Yorkers, with no real fundraising expe-rience. Much of the money they took in during their fund drive each April went toward the next year's fundraising efforts.

Dr. Little surprised Mary by telling her that after Harry Lasker's death, Albert and his sisters had donated $50,000 in their brother's memory. The ASCC had used the interest from this to create their educational pamphlets about cancer's warning signs, which was what had brought the society to Mary's attention in the first place. She acknowledged the usefulness of catching cancer early for greater treatment success. But after more than three decades in exis-tence, she asked Dr. Little, why weren't they looking for ways to prevent cancer's occurrence, or how to stop its progression? He had no answer, so she asked what she could do to help. He was keen to hold a conference, he said, and to publish a book on the status of research into the disease. The cost for the two projects would total $5,000, which Mary gave him.

The doctor then wondered whether Albert would be interested in being on the ASCC board. Mary demurred, but suggested Emerson Foote instead (both of his parents had died of cancer). Foote agreed, and with his business acumen and Mary's drive, in 1944 the society doubled their fundraising take from the year before. Their hard work netted two other notable successes that year. First, with Albert's help, the society's name changed. The new American Cancer Society debuted in October. Second, Mary prevailed on her friend Lois Mattox Miller, a roving editor for *Reader's Digest,* to publish an article in the November 1944 issue. With the title "Fifty Thousand Could Live," it was a plea for people to seek early diagnoses. But it also had a cleverly placed request for donations to ACS. And the money began to flow.

A $1,000 check arrived from a battleship in the Pacific, and an equal amount was sent by radio newsman Walter Winchell. So many envelopes arrived, in fact, that the society's small staff was overwhelmed. Albert was overwhelmed, too, but in a very positive way. He had supported Mary's efforts from afar. Now, seeing her success energized him. He was a major stockholder in the Pepsodent Company, and happened to be in the middle of negotiating the toothpaste company's sale to Unilever. Albert would sell, he told Unilever, *only* if they would make a $50,000 contribution to ACS every year for the next five years. Unilever agreed. Albert took the first check to the ACS office and informed them that 100 percent of it *and* the ensuing checks had to be earmarked for research. ACS agreed as well.

By the start of 1945, however, Mary had become frustrated with the society's disorganization. The fundraising goal that April was $5 million and the clock for publicizing that year's campaign was ticking. She again spoke with her friend Lois Mattox, telling her she was thinking of backing out of the project. The journalist snapped at her, "Are you going to let all the people continue to die, and put off making any real effort to get money for research for another year?" The rebuke lit a fire under Mary. She phoned Dr. Little, telling him that she would hire John Price Jones, head of the country's biggest fundraising company (Jones had purportedly personally raised more than $400 billion), and cover his $80,000 fee. But ACS must agree that 25 percent of everything raised would be set aside for research. The society acquiesced, and Foote went to work organizing a publicity campaign. But then they hit a snag.

Just as the term "birth control" had been taboo to put into print a few years earlier, the word "cancer" couldn't be spoken on the radio. Unlike the prohibition on the term "birth control," however, there was no law against using the word "cancer" in the media; the proscription was merely intended to spare Americans from having to think about it. The disease couldn't be cured; it could scarcely be treated. Why upset listeners by bringing it up? Like Albert before him, though, Emerson Foote was now an enormous purchaser of radio commercial airtime. When reminded of that, and then told what a difference could be made in human lives if more research money was raised, the network heads couldn't resist. On April 28, 1945, the ultra-popular comedy radio show *Fibber McGee and Molly* presented a public service special. For the first time ever, cancer was brought out of the shadows and its name was spoken on air. The fourteen-minute program then ended with an appeal to donate to ACS to help them meet their $5 million goal that year. Donations, McGee said, could be made by mail, addressing the envelope to "cancer," in care of the post office.[7]

For their part, the Mahoneys chaired the 1945 fundraising efforts in Miami, increasing the total brought in from $1,000 in 1944 to $55,000. At the end of the campaign that year, the final figures were astounding: with almost $4.3 million raised, ACS had nearly met its goal.[8] More exciting was that $960,000 would go to research. And what did the federal government plan to spend on cancer research that same year? Five hundred thousand dollars. "This on the number-two killer of people in the United States," Mary remarked incredulously. Then, channeling Albert, she added, "That's not even enough for a good campaign for Pepsodent toothpaste."

As he watched the donations grow, Albert became so enthusiastic, he joined the ACS board. The other members' lethargy shocked him. He, Mary, and Foote agreed that more lay board members were needed. At the next meeting, Albert presented the idea that 50 percent of their number should come from outside the medical field, which would include Mary and Foote. A casual agreement was struck, but when Albert began recruiting other top corporate executives, the doctors on the board balked. Being the consummate salesman he was, Albert persuaded some to his view and, after thanking the others for their service, showed them the door.

The Laskers were thrilled with the success of the ACS fundraising and the direction it appeared the society was heading. But they knew that to achieve their ultimate goal—the conquest of cancer—federal money would still be a necessity. Thankfully, the seeds for that had already been planted.

Claude Denson Pepper was born in 1900, a year after Mary. But his roots in a poor farming family in Chambers County, Alabama, were as far from her privileged midwestern upbringing as could be possible. After graduating from Harvard Law School (he was there while Mary was at Radcliffe, although she didn't know him), Pepper taught briefly at the University of Alabama before moving to tiny Perry, Florida. He served its residents in the state House of Representatives for a single term, and then moved to Tallahassee. In an uncanny turn of events, he found himself a U.S. senator in 1931, after first the elected senator and then his replacement died within a month of each other.

By chance in the spring of 1944, Mary met Pepper at the chic Park Avenue restaurant Voisin. The iconic eatery had appeared in the writings of Ernest Hemingway. But the Lasker-Pepper encounter, while never publicized, had greater consequences. Mary had learned that the senator was chairman of the Subcommittee on Wartime Health and Education. Given that the Allies were making impressive advances in Europe, she was keen to speak with people in Washington about postwar scientific research. Pepper was the perfect place to start.

When Mary shared with Albert her good fortune at meeting Pepper, he suggested they call the Mahoneys. Surely they would know the senator from Florida and could arrange further contact with him. Fortuitously, Pepper was up for reelection. Positive press in the *Miami Daily News* (Dan Mahoney's paper) would be a great reward for his future support of Mary's mission. Learning of the plan, the Mahoneys were on board. And Albert pledged financial support for the senator's reelection campaign. It wasn't an unusual thing; people often paid to enhance their own power by supporting candidates. Albert's offer to do so in the name of medical research, however, was rather rare. As a result of these efforts, two Pepper staff members came to the Laskers' home for tea and a discussion. The senator, they said, was interested in holding hearings on national health. That was all Mary needed to hear.

She gave them a full-blown presentation of what she knew about the state of American medical research, ending with the fact that between $10 million and $15 million had been expended on health research when it mattered to the military. What would happen after the war? The staff members returned to Washington, D.C., armed with Mary's information. It impressed Pepper, and he scheduled hearings on the subject for September 17 and 18. Mary and Florence met in Washington to attend them.

Some of the testimony came from staffers of the Selective Service System, who provided the startling statistic that—in supposedly the healthiest country in the world—40 percent of the American men who had volunteered for military service had been rejected for health reasons. They suffered from conditions that, with adequate treatment gleaned from adequate research, could most likely be alleviated.[9] The two women lunched with Pepper in the Senate Dining Room after the hearings ended. Supported by what had been revealed, they reiterated the dire need for more research. Pepper agreed with them that federal funds were necessary, and on a much larger scale than those currently allocated. It was a new idea to the senator, but he promised more robust hearings on it in December, and asked Mary to send him a list of people who might testify. This was her first assignment in selecting "citizen witnesses."

Mary began combing through her address book, while Albert employed his fifty years of advertising experience by transforming her facts and figures into human perspectives. Aside from the military rejections, statistics showed the mammoth toll of work absenteeism due to illness. It was more costly to industry than anything else, including strikes. In 1944, only 3.5 percent of the total national income went to medical care. Distilling that down, Albert's pitch was perfect: "To keep ourselves from dying, we only spend 3 1/2 percent of what we spend on everything else!"[10]

The first Senate hearings on federal research funding had gone well. But Mary wasn't one to place all of her eggs in a single basket. Her relationship with the White House was another useful basket. She went back to Washington to visit Anna Rosenberg, sharing her hopes that the significant medical research conducted in the past four years would continue in some form after the war. Anna agreed, and asked Mary to write a memorandum on the topic that she could take to the president. FDR was intrigued by the idea and called in Judge Samuel Rosenman for his thoughts. The judge served the president in a number of capacities: speechwriter, senior advisor, and first official White House counsel. He was also a friend of the Laskers. FDR asked Rosenman to write a letter to Vannevar Bush, the engineer and inventor who headed the Office of Scientific Research and Development, asking for recommendations about scientific and medical research in peacetime.

The letter Rosenman wrote, which Roosevelt signed and sent on November 17, 1944, asked Bush to address several questions. Among them were: "With particular reference to the war of science against disease, what can be done now to organize a program for continuing in the future the work which has been done in medicine and related sciences?" "What can the Government do now and in the future to aid research activities by public and private organizations?"[11] While the words came from the president, they echoed Mary's memo verbatim.

She, Albert, and Florence arrived in Washington, D.C., on December 13 for Senator Pepper's second set of hearings, which would begin the next morning. A meeting with his staff members at their Statler Hotel suite had been arranged to discuss how those hearings would play out. Mary's suggested list of witnesses, along with Albert's statistical slug lines, were all carefully choreographed. Mary later reflected, "We were the grassroots rising!" That humble description understates the significance of what they caused to happen. This would be the first time that Congress had ever heard anything this specific about the need for medical research in the United States.

"Medical research has been mobilized for war," Pepper's opening statement began, "and it has contributed magnificently to the coming victory of the United Nations. . . . It appears to me that the Federal Government must ask itself at this time, 'How can the Government participate in the future development of medical research when the emergency is ended?' . . . We have invited outstanding medical investigators here today to give us the benefit of their views on this subject. The nation will listen to their opinions with respect because of their authority in research and because they have the interests of humanity at heart."

Florence and the Laskers would hang on every word as they sat in the hearing room. One of the early witnesses was Dr. Alfred Richards, chairman of the OSRD's Committee on Medical Research. His testimony on the wartime benefits of the committee's work was impressive. His concluding thoughts, however, were significant: "If the concerted efforts of medical investigators which have yielded so much of value during the war are to be continued on any comparable scale during the peace, the conclusion is inescapable that they must be supported by government."

Not long after, Dr. Henry Simms, of the College of Physicians and Surgeons at Columbia University (and a Lasker witness selection), rose to speak. In his opening statement, he said he believed there was unanimous agreement that the present financial support of peacetime medical research was woefully inadequate. The citizen lobbyists' hearts jumped at that statement. Dr. Simms continued that if $10 million was made available the following year (1945), and if the amount was increased progressively until it reached $50 million in 1953 and then was held at that level moving forward, "I believe this could be profitably spent for important research on urgent medical problems."

Dr. Simms's testimony was supplemented with data available from two sources. First, the Medical Memorial Fund (an organization newly formed to ascertain the need for medical research) revealed that in 1940 more than half a million people died of diseases of the heart and arteries. Yet just 17¢ per death had been spent on research. In the cancer column that year, only the equivalent of dinner at an average-priced Washington restaurant had been spent: $2.18 per death ($44 today).

The doctor's second source, he said, was Mrs. Albert D. Lasker. Her data listed the current sufferers of disability in the country, including 3.75 million with heart disease, 1.45 million with mental diseases, and 930,000 with cancer; the total was equivalent to the combined populations of Chicago, Detroit, and Los Angeles. The doctor also brought forth a concept no one had yet mentioned: long-term research. The one- and two-year grants then available were too short, he said, to solve many of the problems, specifically those relating to heart disease. That work would require grants of five to ten years, which in turn would require more money.

At the end of Simms's testimony, Pepper asked the doctor, "Would [it] be a wise expenditure of public funds to aid medical research, and [would] the expenditures of more funds lead to better health and longer life for people of the country?" Dr. Simms responded, "It would be a wise investment." Music to the ears for Mary, Albert, and Florence.

Dr. Rolla Dyer, director of NIH, was soon called to speak. Pepper asked him how much was being appropriated annually to NCI. Dr. Dyer responded that its budget was $560,000, a figure that included building maintenance, utilities, salaries, supplies of all kinds, and so on. Sixteen percent of the budget was spent on research, focused mainly on making patients comfortable. Pepper asked if more funds had ever been requested from Congress, specifically for medical research. Dr. Dyer never used the word "no," but he assured the senator that NCI had always been given what it needed. The doctor was proud to have never asked for more money, which astonished the senator.

In explanation, Dr. Dyer reiterated what Dr. Gregg had told the Laskers two years earlier: "Our trouble is in finding ideas and the men to carry them out." Yet, Pepper pointed out, several of Dyer's fellow witnesses had stated that profitable research *could* be undertaken and that personnel *were* available. Dr. Dyer saw where the questions were heading. After a few more in the same vein, he concluded his contribution to the hearing with a change of direction. Referencing the CMR, he proclaimed that if such an approach had worked during wartime, why not in a time of peace? A wobbly, but nonetheless positive, endorsement.

The last to testify was Dr. Cornelius Rhoads, director of Memorial Hospital for the Treatment of Cancer and Allied Diseases in New York (now known as Memorial Sloan Kettering Cancer Center). At the time of the hearings, Dr. Rhoads was on loan to the U.S. Army as a colonel, working in the OSRD. Mary and Florence had handpicked him as a witness, after having had dinner with him during the September hearings. As many others would do in the future, once the two women pled their case for research, he was on board. Dr. Rhoads's testimony began with the obvious: "If we don't carry on medical research, we won't get medical research done, and we will still have problems that can be solved only by medical research." His answers to Pepper's questions were supportive and valuable, although he was somewhat hampered in his ability to provide detail by the OSRD's need for secrecy.

His last words, however, would be echoed many times in the years to come: "The only opposition I can imagine to the continued federal support of medical research would be by those who would say that this would be a dictatorship, that this would strangle individual initiative."[12]

That fear was based on what the world had just learned. The Nazi government had commandeered many of Europe's top scientists and doctors, forcing them to research what it wanted and telling them how to do it. Mary and Florence took note. Research must be done freely, and that was nonnegotiable.

⟶

While excitement, stress, and disappointment swirled around the citizen lobbyist couple, Albert and Mary Lasker also led a marvelous behind-the-scenes life. Certainly wealth, success, and good looks don't prevent bad things from happening. Mary had spent nine years wed to a man who, for most of that time, was a depressed alcoholic. Albert had experienced the sudden death of a wife he adored and the embarrassment of an ill-conceived second marriage. Yet those heartbreaks prepared them to love each other. And not only was that love strong, but it never got in the way of who each of them was.

Mary's interest in fine art had never wavered, although she still rued the fact that she'd had to sell the small collection she'd begun in the 1920s in order to support her husband, the gallery, and herself during the Depression. Albert, on the other hand, had never developed an interest in art, although he loved things of beauty. He was willing to spend a fortune on flowers and gardens, and had overseen the advertising revolution of adding artwork to ads. But in the world of fine art, he was a neophyte. In 1940, Albert happened to be at the home of a friend who had an immense collection of modern art. There he met Alfred Frankfurter, editor of *Art News* magazine. They would later become great friends, but on that night, as they stood looking at some of the collection, Frankfurter was struck not only by Albert's naivety but also by his courage in exposing his lack of sophistication. Questions flowed forth: Albert wanted to know what the paintings represented, why the artist might have used a particular color or style, and more.

Early on in their relationship, Mary had realized that no one had ever helped Albert become interested in paintings. But it certainly wasn't a deal-breaker for her. "He's marvelous the way he is," she said to herself at the time. "I'm madly in love with him, and I'm not going to try to reform him about paintings. If he doesn't like paintings, I can't help it."

However, they did talk about art. Mary explained how modern art had actually influenced modern industrial design, packaging, magazine layouts, and more. The artists, she said, were really pioneers. Viewing and—even more importantly—owning modern art was akin to buying the first of any other original invention. Perhaps the most important thing she taught Albert was that there was no right or wrong to art. One could love a painting for many reasons; it was very subjective. Albert let all of this sink in for a while.

The Laskers' grand residence at 29 Beekman Place was a majestic brick and limestone town house that had been built by CBS founder William Paley eight years earlier. And like the nearby penthouse where Mary had been living when she met Albert, this home, too, had a view of the East River, and so much more. It was seven stories tall, with each story devoted to just a few rooms, for a total of 10,500 square feet. From the grand foyer flowed a formal dining room seating twenty, with dramatic views of the river seen through the full window wall. Upper floors were accessed by either a winding staircase or an elevator. On the second level, an immense formal drawing room and a library welcomed guests, while Albert and Mary's bedroom suites spread across the third floor. Above that were eight more bedrooms, along with the necessary bathrooms, a laundry, and servants' quarters. As had been the case with all of Albert's other residences, it was breathtaking. And it had a great deal of wall space.

Perusing the newspaper one fall day in 1944, Mary saw that an upcoming auction at Parke-Bernet Galleries would feature Renoir's *Fleurs et Chats* (*Flowers and Cats*), which depicted two kittens playing beneath a large decorative bowl of bright red geraniums. The sale was rather obscure, one Mary thought other collectors might not notice. That could give her the opportunity for a real steal, and she was willing to bid up to $10,000 for the piece. She invited Albert to come along, although, ever the independent, she announced she would use her own money if she bought anything. Albert agreed to join her. It was his first auction, and when he arrived at the gallery, he became somewhat intimidated and told her he'd wait in the hallway. She insisted he join her, and although there weren't seats together, he found one directly behind her.

When the painting came up, Mary began bidding and stopped when it got to $10,000. The next voice she heard was Albert's, behind her. Caught up in the excitement, he continued to bid right up to $25,000. Suddenly, though, fright got the better of him. He'd never bid for a painting in his life and couldn't believe he'd let himself be swept away. What Albert didn't know was that his bidding nemesis was an eminent art dealer who had no intention of stopping until he'd won the painting, which he promptly took to his own gallery three hundred feet up the street.[13]

Not long after the auction, Albert looked at their still relatively bare walls and announced, "What we need around here are some good paintings." To Mary's amazement, he got his hat and left. His destination was the gallery that had won the Renoir. And he came home not only with *Fleurs et Chats* but also with another Renoir of that period: the radiant *La Barque* (*The Boat*). He was thrilled with his negotiated purchase price of $105,000 for the two pieces ($1.7 million today). Mary was aghast, as that seemed like a pretty steep price tag. But two decades later, she had reconsidered her opinion: "In light of present prices," she laughed, "it was one of the great bargains of the world!"

Chapter 5

"Money Is Just Frozen Energy"

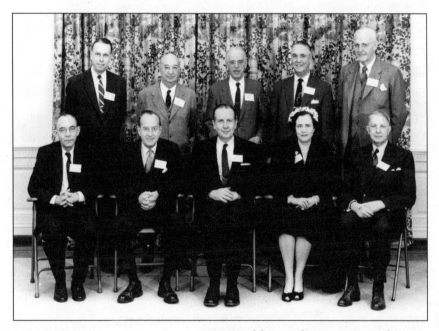

Members of the National Advisory Heart Council, circa 1948.

M ary had gotten to know Franklin and Eleanor Roosevelt on a personal level, although she still didn't think of herself as particularly political. As the 1944 election loomed, she considered voting Republican again. But the party's platform was too conservative for her. Although the Republican candidate, Thomas Dewey, did better against FDR than any of his previous three opponents had, the president would remain in the White House for a fourth term. And both Laskers had voted for him. Mary attended the inauguration on Saturday, January 20, 1945, as Anna's guest. Due to World War II austerity measures, the inauguration was held on the South Portico of the White House, rather than at the Capitol. The traditional parade down Pennsylvania Avenue to the White House had been canceled as well. But Mary and Anna had been invited to join one hundred or so people in the East Room after the ceremony. A sparse lunch was served, and they chatted with both Mrs. Roosevelt and the new Second Lady, Bess Truman. The president made the rounds, greeting his guests, but then retired to his own rooms.

A month later, Roosevelt attended the week-long Yalta Conference, along with British prime minister Winston Churchill and Soviet premier Joseph Stalin. Their meeting in the resort town on the stormy Black Sea was to discuss how the world would be divided once the war was over. When FDR returned to Washington, those who knew him were shocked at how thin and frail he looked. On April 12, he was in Warm Springs, Georgia—a favorite destination—sitting for a portrait. Roosevelt said to the artist, "I have a terrific pain in the back of my head," and then slumped forward in his chair, unconscious. His doctor was summoned, and he diagnosed a massive intracerebral hemorrhage. A few hours later, Franklin Delano Roosevelt was dead at the age of sixty-three.[1] Mary was saddened on a number of levels, not the least of which was that his death reminded her of the deaths of her parents.

By this time, her voracious newspaper clipping and brochure gathering had become an obsession. The more Mary learned about the state of health research, the angrier she got. People were suffering because of a lack of education, on the part of both patients and the scientific community. She created a list of four topics she felt were priorities. First were heart disease and cancer. As had been brought out during the 1944 Pepper hearings, those two diseases killed more Americans every year than all other causes of death combined. Next was mental illness, which incapacitated people in every aspect of their lives; the problem now compounded by the number of men returning from the war who were suffering from battle fatigue (what we now know as post-traumatic stress disorder). Lastly, Mary felt some form of national health insurance was critical. As a woman of wealth, she could afford the best treatment available for any disease. But for many Americans, illness meant one of two choices: either get better on their own or die.

It wasn't just the distress at suffering and untimely deaths that drove Mary. It was money. Being sick was a drain on all of America. "It's an economy to find new treatments and cures for the major cripplers and killers of the people of the United States," she proclaimed. "If people are able to stay in good health, they produce goods and earn income, which in turn gets back to the federal treasury in the form of taxes."

Having Florence as a friend in this fight was a blessing. There weren't many (if any) other lobbyists in Washington who had their altruistic motives. Plus, Capitol Hill lobbying was a "good old boys" affair; there were no other women. But while Florence had the same research interests as Mary, they had differing views on the type of medical research that should be funded. Florence favored *basic* research, which focuses on advancing knowledge. Mary, on the other hand, was a strong advocate of *applied* research, which directs its efforts toward finding a solution to a specific problem. Her personal connection to deadly diseases propelled her to demand faster cures. At the end of the day, however, Mary and Florence brought myriad complementary skills to the table. And the companionship that each provided the other amid all the difficulties of presenting such new—and, as some thought, strange—concepts was invaluable.

"If I'd been alone," Mary said, "people would have thought I was a solitary nut. It was more unusual for there to be two nuts [together] than one!"

But it was Albert who was Mary's greatest ally. He had been attracted to her charm, intelligence, and drive. Now, coupled with his connections and vast wealth, her mission could be accelerated. Albert wasn't interested in *how* things got done. Rather, his interest was in getting results for things he knew *should* get done. Seeing what could happen with a project if enough money was available to support it excited him. It was how he had built his one-of-a-kind success in advertising. He saw Mary as the "volunteer citizen lobbyist," and he was willing to help her achieve her goals. "Without him," Mary later said, "nothing could have been done."

In Washington, D.C., an uncountable number of ideas are exchanged every day. It's no surprise, then, that often several people are concurrently working on the same issue. After Pepper's hearings the previous December had concluded, and at the urging of Mary and Florence, the Florida senator had introduced a bill to create the National Medical Research Foundation. Meanwhile, Vannevar Bush's recommendations for a peacetime version of OSRD (the proposal FDR had requested as a result of Mary's memo) were released in July 1945 in a report entitled "Science: The Endless Frontier." Bush also suggested a new federal research organization: the National Science Foundation (NSF). To get that ball rolling, Senator Harley Kilgore, a West Virginia Democrat, along with Democrat Warren Magnuson, introduced a bill officially asking Congress to support its creation.

Pepper's bill met with resistance on a number of fronts, so it seemed to him that the sensible thing to do was to jump ship and join his bill with Kilgore and Magnuson's, which he did without telling Mary and Florence. They liked the idea of a new and separate research entity, since it was very clear that those in existence—the Public Health Service and NIH—weren't moving quickly enough to solve anything. But they were surprised and disappointed at Pepper's desertion, compounded by the fact that, within the proposed NSF bill, medical research would become only one of four scientific categories to get attention. That, they feared, would relegate medical research to the back seat once again. Further distressing to their cause was the growing division between politicians, scientists, and the medical community on whether the wartime medical research effort should even continue in peacetime.

The two women were quickly learning the complexities of the legislative process. Politicians supported research in fits and starts; sometimes their north star was whatever personal experiences they had had with diseases, but more often it was whatever was popular among their constituents. And while they had been polite to Mary and Florence, the fact was that women—and their opinions—were rarely included in high-powered decision-making scenarios. Less than 2 percent of the House of Representatives was female, and the first woman U.S. senator wouldn't be elected without filling another senator's seat until Nancy Kasse-baum in 1978 (although she began her term eleven days early as her predecessor resigned prior to the end of his term).

Within the halls and laboratories of science and medicine, other challenges were developing. Scientists who had gladly stepped up when asked to help achieve military victory, and who were more than adequately compensated for their work, were suddenly distrustful of any government involvement in science after the war. And the same public officials who had benefited from scientific successes were now expressing reciprocal distrust in the scientific community's ability to handle significant research funding. Egos and conflicting personal beliefs have long been a part of human society. Everyone, especially those with a modicum of power, protects his little corner of the world.

Upon assuming his new duties, President Harry Truman asked Judge Rosenman (who was now holding the same positions for Truman as he had for FDR) which of FDR's projects had not been achieved. "I want to carry out everything that Roosevelt intended to do," Truman explained. Rosenman told him that just before his last inauguration, FDR had promised to present a health message to Congress. (It had been Mary who suggested it to him.) Truman asked Rosenman to draft a message, and the judge asked Mary to come to Washington in May 1945 to talk details.

The first draft of the message was exceedingly good, Mary told Rosenman. But, she pointed out, there was no reference to the need for more research in the field of mental illness. The judge added it, and then passed the revised draft along to the president. Mary had hoped to meet with Truman during the same Washington visit to thank him for his support of American health, and, probably more importantly, to encourage him to deliver the health message as soon as possible. The president was unable to see her, however. He had just received news that the Nazis had surrendered, and the White House was a hive of activity. Three months later, the Japanese stopped fighting, too, although the official signing of the surrender didn't take place until September 2. World War II was finally over. Consequently, it wasn't until September 8 that President Truman could finally receive Mrs. Albert Lasker in the Oval Office.

Her plan was to chat about the still undelivered health message, but Truman had other things on his mind. She could see he was uncomfortable about becoming president. His vice presidency had been short (just eighty-two days), and during that period he had been more or less sidelined. Truman had met privately with Roosevelt only a few times. He had never been in the Oval Office and had never been told about the construction of the atomic bomb. When presented with its existence, the move to actually use it was not an easy one for Truman. He later admitted, "It was the hardest decision I ever had to make."

At the very start of their meeting, Mary sensed his unease. "I could see that this was so much on his mind because he was still justifying himself, out loud to a complete stranger. He said, 'You know by doing this [using the atomic bombs at Hiroshima and Nagasaki], [Secretary of Defense George] Marshall told me we saved the lives of 300,000 American men, because that many men would have been killed in the landings on Japan.'" It had been just a month since the cities had been bombed.

"He felt very tentative and apologetic about being president," Mary went on. "This seemed so extraordinary, because I came to the highest officer of the land to get something done about the health of people. I was taking him for granted. But he was excusing himself."

As would become her trademark, Mary had respectful yet succinct talking points to share with the president. She gently redirected the conversation, asking him if he would move ahead with the health message to Congress. It would be a historic event, she told him, as he would be the first president in history to take an interest in the health of the people. This appealed to Truman on a number of levels. During his days as a county judge, he had seen many poor rural families who lacked money for medical care.

"Will you do it?" Mary asked him.

"Yes, I'll do it," Truman replied.

Truman also agreed to announce that he favored national health insurance, and that would be historic for a sitting president as well. It would also be very daring, and politically very dangerous. After further consideration, he called Rosenman and suggested that perhaps some preplanned and carefully placed citizen support for both the health message and national insurance would ensure that those proposals would be better received. Judge Rosenman passed along to Mary the president's request for a citizens group.

Mary wasted no time organizing the Committee on National Health. She felt that formal committees, with a board of esteemed names, would give her work legitimacy. Although the names varied, it was a practice she would continue throughout her career. Mary asked her sister, Alice (who had married architect Allmon "Al" Fordyce in 1939), to be secretary of the committee, which also included Anna, Henry Kaiser (a famed shipbuilder who created a revolutionary health care program for his employees), Gardner Cowles (founder of Cowles Media Company), the Mahoneys, Dan Mahoney's former father-in-law, James Cox, and former First Lady Eleanor Roosevelt. Albert offered to fund advertising in the *New York Times,* the *Washington Post,* and the *Washington Star.*

Truman delivered his health message to Congress on November 19, 1945. The following week, Mrs. Roosevelt's recurring newspaper column, "My Day," began with this sentence: "I have signed today an endorsement of President Truman's health message."[2] Mary would have been justified in thinking that, of all people, the widow of one of the most popular presidents in history would be able to move the needle in favor of the message's content. But she hadn't counted on powerful opposition from the American Medical Association (AMA).

"The physicians of this country will not be regimented!" Dr. Herman Kretchmer, the AMA's president, declared in a newspaper article hastily assembled to present the AMA's opposition to the proposals. Kretchmer went on, "It should be perfectly clear to every one that regimentation always leads to totalitarianism." He foresaw "chaos in medical care" and "socialized medicine" if the country followed through with Truman's suggestions.[3] The AMA might have been surprised by the novel ideas coming out of Washington this time, but its opposition to such plans would be far better organized in the future.

Mary was shocked at the AMA's response. She had had no idea that creating a new research entity—such as was proposed by the bill before Congress—and offering a new way of viewing health care would turn out to be such an immense task. Perhaps, she thought, it would be less of a climb to light a fire under those within NIH. When 1946 dawned, Mary and Florence tentatively took that approach. And they simultaneously learned that heart disease and cancer weren't the only conditions being considered by Congress for research funding.

Just as birth control and cancer made people squeamish, discussions of mental health were also taboo in the middle of the twentieth century. In the December 1944 Pepper hearings, however, Mary had made certain it would come to light by recommending that Dr. George Stevenson, medical director of the National Committee on Mental Hygiene, be included on the witness list. In his opening statement, Dr. Stevenson revealed that the wartime medical rejection rate for military enlistees included not just those disqualified for physical conditions but also those disqualified for mental ones. Some called it a "national disgrace," he explained, while he preferred to think of the revelation as a "national problem."

"The rate of rejections and discharges from the armed services has shown," Stevenson said in his testimony, "how serious are the limitations of our mental health and how we will have to busy ourselves to reduce these limitations."[4]

By the next year, Tennessee Democratic congressman Percy Priest had learned so much about the needs of returning military personnel that he introduced a bill to establish a mental health division within PHS. Among other things, it would provide training for psychiatrists, who were in shorter supply than any other medical specialty. When Mary and Florence heard about Priest's bill, they immediately called on Pepper to introduce similar legislation in the Senate. As they made the rounds, speaking to senators about the importance of mental research, one said to them, "Don't talk to us about crazy people!"[5] Not long afterward, however, that senator heard about a colleague's son who had committed suicide, and he changed his tune about the mental health bill.

The Laskers hosted dinner parties to talk up the legislation. They were such a successful tool in achieving results that Mary would employ them in varying forms the rest of her life. The Mahoneys saw to it that the *Miami Daily News* covered the 1946 hearings, as did the *Washington Post*. The mental health bill passed the House and then the Senate, and was signed into law by President Truman on July 3. The bill approved $17 million to be spent on research grants, psychiatric education, and—best of all—the creation of the National Institute of Mental Health (NIMH), which would become one of several components under the umbrella of NIH. It would also make the name plural, becoming the National Institutes of Health.

Mary and Florence were over the moon. Not only had they been successful, but now they had a road map they could use to guide their other projects through Congress. Shortly after the bill's approval, when Washington insiders asked the women how much money had been appropriated for the new institute, they proudly named the figure, $17 million. Wasn't that merely the amount authorized? they were asked. The women were confused by that second question.

"If a bill mentioned an authorization," Mary later said, "[we thought] that was tantamount to having the money. We were so naive. We found that that [authorization] is one thing, but to get the money was a different matter. You had to go to entirely different people and that was another world." A lesson was learned.

Mary was also learning about the enormous juggling act required of a citizen lobbyist. A great many congressional hearings and meetings had to be conducted before any significant legislation could pass. She and Florence attended as many as they could, supplementing them with visits to the offices of important legislators. They went to medical meetings around the country, too, and spoke to experts. Mary devoured newspapers and reports over coffee when she arose, and could still be found with papers and journals spread around her at bedtime.

The reading aside, away from the Washington fray, Mrs. Albert Lasker enjoyed all the benefits that came with that moniker. And, oh, the fun the Laskers had! In the months prior to their annual spring Florida trips, they made a pilgrimage to the famous La Quinta Hotel, forty-five acres snugged up against the pink-hued Santa Rosa Mountains, twenty-five miles from Palm Springs, California. There they rented an adobe bungalow and hobnobbed with Hollywood stars and titans of industry. To further escape the noise, dirt, and cold temperatures of New York, together with the Mahoneys they bought the Z Triangle Ranch in Kirkland, Arizona. Florence later laughed about Albert, the dapper city dweller, not quite transitioning to the rugged rancher. But he was always a good sport about it.[6]

Regardless of where they were—except, perhaps, at the remote Z Triangle Ranch—there were always parties and dinners to host and attend. They collected friends and acquaintances for the pure pleasure of knowing them: actors, writers, statesmen, scientists, artists, even royalty. Things slowed down a bit when Albert was struck with a severe health issue. He developed a staph infection and was given penicillin (a relatively new drug), but the infection was resistant, causing him to be hospitalized off and on for seven months. Late in 1946, his doctors decided it was bronchial pneumonia and changed his treatment regimen, and he gradually regained strength. Mary fussed over him the entire time, feeling as if half of her were missing if he wasn't standing beside her.

Once the pneumonia was gone, Albert went back to work behind the scenes, always ensuring publicity for Mary's causes. During one of their La Quinta visits, Albert arranged interviews for Mary and Anna, who was visiting. The two women traveled 135 miles west to speak with reporters. Mary was interviewed for the *Los Angeles Times* women's section and was quoted as saying, "It's up to women to see that medical research is accelerated if we don't want to freeze treatment of disease at its present level." She went on, "While 248,000 Americans [were] killed in World War II, during the same four years, more than 600,000 Americans died of cancer alone, to say nothing of the toll taken by heart disease."

Mary pointed out that the "speedy research" done during the war had provided the troops with penicillin and sulfa drugs, along with medications to fend off malaria and other tropical diseases. She knew that the newspaper offered her a much larger stage for those points than the floor of Congress had been. And public interest would move those senators and representatives. The article continued by highlighting Mary's point that peacetime scientific research could, if given support, conquer many diseases, and that the first step in that direction was financial support of laboratories. A quote from Mary ended the article with a call to action: "It will be well for women to study health legislation and to prod their Congressmen to vote for the bills," referring to the four health bills before Congress.[7]

Meanwhile, Anna was interviewed for an article in another section of the newspaper that would address the topic of veterans' aid. With a photo of her wearing one of her signature hats—really, just a mass of little white flowers—the article began rather condescendingly, given its somber topic: "Mrs. Anna Rosenberg, a sharp-eyed little woman . . ." After that, however, the article got serious, telling of the need for support for veterans. It ended by mentioning that Anna was Mary's guest while in California, and that the two of them were next headed to Washington to testify before congressional committees considering national health legislation.[8] This gave them an aura of importance.

Albert also encouraged Mary to think bigger when it came to her research asks. In business, he had never been interested in speaking with anyone who wanted to spend less than a million dollars on their advertising campaign. And his experience on the Shipping Board, Albert explained to Mary, had shown him that senators and representatives were accustomed to dealing with large appropriations. They simply hadn't considered that kind of money in connection to medical research. Mary was a willing student. His input resulted in a question she posed often to scientists and politicians alike: if $15 million wasn't too much to spend advertising tobacco annually (the amount Lucky Strike cigarettes was spending with Lord and Thomas in 1942, when Albert retired), how could $15 million be too much to spend researching the diseases that were killing Americans? (The link between smoking and lung cancer had not yet been confirmed, and would not be until after Albert's death in 1952.)

As Mary and Florence traveled around Washington, shaking hands and delivering their pitches, more and more legislators began to realize that medical research might, indeed, deserve the same kind of substantial funds that roads, the military, and education received. Why, then, did it seem such an uphill battle with the medical community? The Laskers surmised that, for the most part, the era's doctors were small businessmen, with small-business budgets. Many of those who worked at PHS and ACS thought it was madness to ask for the sums Mary was after; the amounts were so stupendous, they thought that she would never be able to get them. Mary wondered if perhaps it was the responsibility of managing so much money that frightened them.

There was another kernel of wisdom Mary gleaned from Albert. "Money is just frozen energy, my husband always said," she explained. "It's the use of money that unfreezes its energy; then things get done." And Mary wanted things done.

—

Mary's zeal for medical research might have ignited Senator Pepper's interest, but Senator Matthew Neely's enthusiasm about combating and curing cancer hadn't lost its flame since his original push in the 1920s and 1930s, when it resulted in NCI. Neely had left the Senate in 1941 to serve as governor of his state. He returned to Congress as a representative in 1945 and brought with him a new cancer bill, which Pepper was happy to sponsor in the Senate. It was simple: Neely asked for the federal government to put up $100 million to be spent as promisingly as possible on cancer. As his bill was discussed on the House floor, he questioned Dr. Dyer (still the head of NIH) about adding to the research budget. Dr. Dyer said the $1.75 million NIH had requested for cancer research was all that could be used.

In response, Neely proclaimed in his dramatic style, "The cancer people have developed a defeatist attitude! If we had fiddled along with the atomic bomb on $1.5 million or $2 million, how long do you suppose we would have been in solving that problem?"

"It would have been a long time," Dr. Dyer responded quietly.[9]

In the gallery, Mary and Florence were enthralled, and sometimes even moved to tears. They were convinced that *this* would be the bill to push research forward. And they weren't alone. Albert thought so, too, and then got the ACS board behind the bill as well. But the question of who would direct the research intervened. The Laskers and the ACS board were still in favor of a separate cancer research organization, staffed by eager scientists who would surely outpace those moving more slowly at NIH. And then, before the vote on the bill, a new version of it appeared. In this one, the $100 million Neely was requesting would remain within the charge of NIH, the very organization whose director didn't see the need for more money. It was a trip through Alice's looking glass, where everything is backward. The Laskers and ACS withdrew support for the legislation.

But it was not all a lost cause. The following year, having pondered the idea of "big money," NIH asked Congress to increase its overall budget. That increase would ultimately take them from less than $8 million in fiscal 1947 to over $26 million by fiscal 1948. In addition, the unsuccessful Neely cancer bill gave Mary the idea of proposing a similar scenario for heart disease research. Unbelievably, no NIH money had ever been designated to study the family of heart diseases, the number one killer in America. And there was only $500,000 available for it from private foundations. As had been the case with cancer, patients and doctors alike looked at the disease and its associated deaths as God's will, something to be accepted. This was an intolerable position as far as Mary was concerned. She was convinced millions of lives could be saved if NIH had a heart institute.

In February 1947, on the way to visit Albert's daughter Frances Brody and her family in California, Mary drew up a draft heart research bill and mailed it to Pepper. The 1946 elections had given control of the Senate to the Republicans. Pepper, a Democrat, was no longer chair of any committee, and he had lost his magic wand as far as the growth of medical research went. Nonetheless, the senator was happy to present the bill (asking for the $100 million), and he suggested a new ally to help them move it through the Senate. Styles Bridges, a Republican from New Hampshire, now controlled the Appropriations Committee and thus the congressional purse strings. Research into heart disease might intrigue Bridges, Pepper thought, particularly since he had suffered a heart attack four months earlier.

When Mary went to see Bridges in April, he was definitely interested. It might have been her smile; it didn't dazzle but warmed, charming Republicans and Democrats alike. He promised a deficiency appropriation hearing (a fancy term for a proceeding that might net a little seed money) to get the research ball rolling. Could she assemble a list of appropriate witnesses? Of course she could, and they would be prepped with her newly born Big Fact Book. Prepared by her National Health Education Committee, a product of the Lasker Foundation, the book included every scintilla of information available concerning the major causes of Americans' death and disability. It would be continually updated, its facts and figures becoming the basis for the next three decades of Congressional testimony that Mary would ignite. If witnesses were anxious about speaking without the necessary stats to back them up, a little studying of the Big Fact Book was very emboldening.

At this juncture, the American Heart Association was very much in the same state as ACS had been when Mary had first become involved: doctors with good intentions, but no sense of how to grow their cause. Armed with Big Fact Book statistics, a number of those doctors were happy to speak before Congress at Bridges's hearing. And that, in turn, paved the way for a larger bill to be presented. Mary turned to NCI director Dr. Leonard Scheele for help in drafting it, since he had been instrumental in the Neely cancer bill. The heart bill proposed a new institute that would provide research grants, along with the creation of an advisory council that would consist of both doctors *and* laypeople. That last stipulation was pure Lasker; ACS provided proof that the strategy of including non-doctors worked.

Mary and Pepper went to Bridges's office in late January 1948 to ask him to sponsor the bill. Bridges said he would, but made what would be a most valuable suggestion. "Don't tie yourself down to any specific amount of money," he told them. "[It] will frighten the boys off from voting for the legislation. If you get the legislation passed, I'll see that you get the money to start, and adequate funds [to continue]."

A similar Lasker-inspired bill had already passed in the House. Mary had been asked to testify for it, which she did. And she hated it. "I find that other people can do it much better and I don't need to," she later said. "Besides, the Congressmen and Senators like to hear from doctors because they think they may get a little free advice. One time a Senator had a long conversation with one of the doctors about the health of his dog!" She never testified again.

On June 10, 1948, the National Heart Act passed, creating the National Heart Institute. All that remained was to get the signature of President Truman, which Mary thought would be a simple formality. But it turned out not to be so simple: an error had resulted in a one-word difference in the text between the House and Senate versions of the bill. That correction had to be made before it went to the president, and the bill languished on a desk as it awaited the change. The clock was ticking toward the end of the fiscal year on June 30 and the annual congressional summer recess. Mary feared that if the bill was put off until Congress reconvened in the fall, the enthusiasm for it might wane. The bill could get shuffled behind others, or potentially tabled altogether.

Meanwhile, as 1948 was a presidential election year, Truman had left Washington to cross the country on a whistle-stop train tour, ending in San Francisco. When the bill was ready for his signature, his constant movement made catching up to him nearly impossible. Leapfrogging over the train by air would be the only way. Truman's political advisor David Niles had remained in Washington to work on other parts of the campaign. He was put aboard the last flight to San Francisco that would make it in time. Mary and Florence sent wires to everyone they knew aboard the train, urging them to be on the lookout for Niles and his precious cargo.

The bill finally made it to Truman on June 16. When he signed it, everyone drew a sigh of relief. Money had still not been appropriated for the National Institute of Mental Health. But Bridges had delivered on his promise of appropriations for the National Heart Institute, and the National Institutes of Health was now truly plural. However, in the bill's final version, only a disappointing $500,000 was allocated for research. Mary's work often seemed as fragile as a sandcastle, tall and strong until a taller and stronger wave washes it away. Yet every step, no matter how small, provided other, sometimes unseen gems.

In this case, the first gem had its genesis in dental work that Albert had had done the year before. As frequently happened when Albert discovered something new, he became fascinated by the field. He learned that dental problems, particularly when they involved infections, were associated with heart problems, likely because of bacteria finding their way from the mouth into the bloodstream and ultimately to the heart. Consequently, Albert had urged that the heart bill also include creation of the National Dental Institute as its own entity, and appropriations had been approved for it as well.

The second gem involved a shift in personnel. Although NIH had its own director, as did each of the institutes that were a part of it, NIH was still an entity within the Public Health Service, which was overseen by the nation's surgeon general. President Truman was impressed with NCI director Scheele's willingness to help draft a bill not directly linked to his own work, and he promoted Scheele to surgeon general. While Scheele's predecessor had merely tolerated calls from Mary and Florence (much as NIH director Dyer did), Scheele made himself highly accessible. That change gave the women confidence that NIH—and not an outside entity—could and should be *the* national home for medical research.

And the last gem gave Mary a new "job." The National Heart Act had also created the National Advisory Heart Council. The roster of its revolutionary inclusion of lay individuals listed Mary as the first non-scientist, and the only woman.

—

Just as Mary was an outsider in Washington when she began her research campaign, Harry Truman was also an outsider when he suddenly became president, despite his having lived in the city since becoming vice president. Unlike Mary, however, who had been to the White House a number of times, dining with the Roosevelts and even spending the night, Truman was as unfamiliar with the presidential residence as he was with the job in general.

In addition, Mrs. Truman wasn't a fan of the lack of privacy that came with politics. And now, as First Lady, that problem was magnified. When Mary first met Bess Truman, she immediately sensed a shyness in her. Florence added the observation that Mrs. Truman was loath to give an opinion, afraid of being poorly judged. She gave a press conference soon after Truman became president and informed the press corps that it would be her one and only. They didn't need to know her, she said. She was not the president. Nor had she been immediately on board with the idea of the president running for his own term in 1948. Like Mary with Albert, however, Bess Truman adored her husband. And she did not want him to be remembered only as an accidental commander in chief.

Thomas Dewey had again been nominated by the Republican Party as their 1948 candidate. He appeared to have such a resounding lead on election night,

Tuesday, November 2, that Truman went to bed without knowing the outcome of the voting. The *Chicago Tribune* even printed papers early on November 3 with the headline "Dewey Defeats Truman." But the man from Missouri wasn't leaving the White House just yet.

That pleased Mary. She had come to respect President Truman, both for his demeanor and for his willingness to listen to her concerns about the nation's health. Despite continued wrath from the AMA, he had delivered a second health message the previous year, 1947. Although it was largely a restatement of the first one, it reemphasized the fact that the president was interested in the field, and it gave the concept of health legislation some currency. Mary was grateful for both of those outcomes. But every morning when she awoke, the knowledge that millions of Americans would suffer that day only propelled her to work harder.

Chapter 6

~

"Can I Help You?"

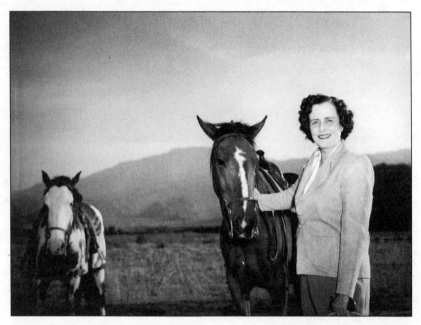

Mary with her horses in Arizona, circa 1940s.

The population of the United States in 1948 was 152,271,417. That year, approximately 1,452,454 of those citizens would die. Some form of heart disease would be the cause of death for 36.9 percent (535,956), and cancer would kill another 14.5 percent (210,606).[1] More alarming than the fact that those two causes alone were responsible for half the nation's deaths was that deaths from both causes were on the rise, in particular cancer deaths, which had doubled since the beginning of the century. These statistics were constantly on Mary's mind. She made sure they, and figures for other illnesses, were on the minds of members of Congress and the president, too. She wouldn't lift her foot off that pedal for a single second.

After attending President Truman's inauguration on a sunny January day in 1949, Mary had gone to Senator Pepper asking him to introduce an arthritis and rheumatism bill. She told him that her much-loved grandfather had suffered from the crippling disease, and she explained that little research was being done on behalf of the seven and a half million Americans currently tortured by it. Clearly, NIH should have a dedicated institute, she said. Pepper agreed and promised to introduce a bill. Her next stop was Representative Percy Priest's office, asking for a companion act to be presented in the House. He, too, concurred that there was a need. The legislators each drew up a bill written identically to the heart bill of 1948.

Mary's trips to Capitol Hill had not gone unnoticed. Seeing her success with NIH, others had begun to propose similar bills, requesting institutes dedicated to multiple sclerosis, cerebral palsy, epilepsy, and other conditions. News of the crowded legislative field now confronting Congress prompted Dr. Norman Topping, then assistant surgeon general, to openly oppose adding more institutes, claiming that the administration of them all would be too complicated. "Personally," Mary sniffed indignantly, "I thought [they] were not half as complicated as the sufferings of the people who had the diseases. The Public Health Service was not terribly motivated by the anxieties about human sufferings; they just didn't want to have too much trouble."

To satisfy all the requests, a twofold solution was conceived. First, the Pepper-led Senate committee would group the bills, creating two institutes: the National Institute of Arthritis and Metabolic Diseases, and the National Institute of Neurological Diseases and Blindness. Although no one in Mary's life had been blind, a group had approached her with facts about how little research was being done for the condition. She was, of course, immediately sympathetic. However, she needed enhanced House support, so she telephoned Wisconsin representative Andrew Biemiller, who was in charge of the appropriate committee. After chatting about her Watertown roots, she asked if he would introduce a bill for the creation of a blindness institute. Without hesitation, Biemiller agreed—a new and surprising phenomenon for Mary, as she had grown accustomed to overcoming dozens of hurdles for each request. "Well, you sound very cooperative, Andy," she told him. "How do you happen to be so interested?" He replied simply, "My mother was blind."

Albert had taught her that "to sell anybody anything, you have to find out what he wants and then help him get it." Mary's goal was to sell Congress on the benefits of health education and research. Given the health statistics she carried around in her head and handbag, she was certain that every senator and representative would eventually know someone with one of the diseases her institutes would research. The way to achieve her goal was simply a question of finding the right person in Congress and offering to help them and those they cared about.

"'Can I help you?' is very powerful if it is meant," Mary later confirmed.

Once the idea to combine the medical conditions into the two new institutes was agreed upon, they were neatly packaged into a massive omnibus bill. The bill also included the provision that the surgeon general—still Dr. Scheele—had the authority to create new institutes. As the months passed, the bill began making its way through both houses of Congress and was eventually signed by the president. Nearly simultaneously, the National Institute of Mental Health finally received its appropriation (the money Mary and Florence had thought existed when the institute was approved in 1946). All of this prompted some to quip that there was "disease of the month" legislating going on.[2] Nonetheless, NIH was now home to six magnificent research facilities whose work would transform the health of America and the world.

Albert had the rare gift of getting younger as he got older. He had become a joyful man, and joy is always a strong tonic. Meeting Mary—twenty years his junior—and being exposed to her exciting projects and interests no doubt played a part. This was no more in evidence than in his continually growing appetite for art. Henri Matisse had become a favorite, and while visiting the artist's studio in Nice in 1949 (a high point of Albert's life, then sixty-nine years long), he told Matisse he wished he were a little younger. The artist, who was eighty, patted Albert's knee paternally and said, "You are still a child." Albert then asked him who the best young artist was in France. "*Moi!*" Matisse replied.[3]

On May 1, 1950, Albert would turn seventy. He decided to forgo his usual party at the Ritz in New York and celebrate in Paris, so he and Mary sailed for the Continent aboard the *Queen Mary*. Both of Albert's daughters and their husbands (Mary and Leigh Block, and Frances and Sidney Brody) accompanied them, along with Albert's two sisters, and good friends Danny Kaye and his wife. The partying rarely stopped in the City of Lights, nor did the antics. On a day trip to Versailles, and at the advice of the curator, Albert and Danny climbed the palace roof for the best view of the gardens.[4] The next day, he and Mary strolled the Champs-Elysées, interspersing glasses of wine with gallery combing. The Blocks and Brodys had become art collectors as well.

In the midst of all this, Albert announced he wanted to make a trip to the newly created state of Israel, inviting his sisters to go along. He had given $50,000 the previous year for the establishment of a children's clinic in Jerusalem. Albert was neither for or against Zionism, yet he felt this was his ancestral land, and he wanted to see the clinic. It would be an eighteen-day trip. He and Mary had never been separated for more than a few days during their ten years of marriage, and while they were apart, Albert wrote her beautiful love letters. "It is good consolation," he penned, "being so far away for so long to confirm to myself how much your companionship means to me."[5]

Meanwhile, Anna Rosenberg had arrived in Paris to keep Mary company. They scoured more galleries and selected eight paintings they thought Albert would like, figuring he'd pick out one or two. When Mary wired what she'd found, Albert wrote, "Darling, as to the paintings, . . . use your own judgement to buy what you think we should, and pay what is right. . . . I leave it to you, knowing you will make the right decision."[6]

This was a surprise. Although Mary had been Albert's art tutor, he had his own opinions. Not long before their trip to Paris, in fact, she had purchased Picasso's *Still Life with Fish*, which she loved. But when it was delivered to Beekman

Place, Albert detested it. The painting was relegated to an out-of-the-way corridor in their home. As a further insult to the painting, Albert affixed a note to its back: "This picture belongs to Mary Lasker and is not to be thought of as part of the Albert Lasker Collection." Now, however, when Albert returned to Paris from Israel, he bought all eight paintings that Mary had selected, several of which were Picassos.

Before the birthday partying broke up and they sailed for home, Albert learned that *Le Zouave*, van Gogh's painting of a French North African soldier, was available. He had seen pictures of it and really wanted it. But it was in Switzerland, and he didn't feel like making the trip. Albert also heard that a Brazilian millionaire was interested in the painting; ever the competitor, he didn't want to miss out. So he had the piece shipped by rail to Paris on approval. When it arrived, he and Mary went to the customs office at the Gare de Lyon to see it. The lighting in the office was poor, so it was carried out into the sunlight. Albert loved it and bought it right there on the street for $85,000 ($1 million in today's money).[7]

The Laskers returned home in June, and almost immediately two significant wars began. The seeds of the first war were planted in 1945 at the Yalta Conference in anticipation of the end of World War II. At the time, the Soviet Union already occupied the northern part of the Korean Peninsula, so the landmass was divided at the thirty-eighth parallel, with the Allies occupying the southern part. In the ensuing years, the North and South developed governments in accordance with their occupiers, and the north became Communist. Clashes began occurring on their mutual border. Then at dawn on Saturday, June 25, 1950, the northern forces invaded, and the Korean War began.

The second war would have far greater consequences for the Laskers. At the end of 1949, Albert had complained of abdominal discomfort. A thorough going-over, including X-rays, revealed nothing out of the ordinary. Once his birthday trip was over, he again had abdominal upset, but figured it was probably due to the rich food he'd consumed abroad. However, when things hadn't changed by the first of July, Albert checked into the Harkness Pavilion (reserved for private patients) at Columbia-Presbyterian Medical Center.

He underwent exploratory surgery on July 5, and more extensive surgery a week later. A tumor in Albert's colon was discovered, which was removed along with a cluster of nearby lymph nodes. When lab results came back a few weeks later, the diagnosis was cancer. Mary became more desperate than ever to step up research on the disease. She also knew how much Albert *hated* discussions of illness, *hated* being sick himself, and, given the death of his brother, Harry, *hated* cancer. She decided that telling him the diagnosis wouldn't stop the disease, and his distress might make matters worse. Aside from the doctors and two other people, Mary kept the cancer news to herself, and prayed it had been caught in time.

⟿

Although it came in as runner-up to heart disease in terms of the number of annual deaths, cancer was the most feared disease on the planet in 1950. It conjured up images of slow and agonizing demise, bereaved spouses, and orphaned children. The very word invoked the terror of untimely death. It was spoken of in hushed tones, and it was never discussed in public. The notion of sickly, skeletal, and surgery-maimed individuals was too much for people to think about. So they didn't.

While more was being learned about cancer all the time, researchers were still in the dark as to why normal cells suddenly begin to grow uncontrollably. In other words, why cells became cancer—which was the basis of knowing how to cure it—was a complete mystery. That meant a very poor prognosis for those with the disease, illustrated by a twenty-cent booklet published jointly in 1947 by ACS and NCI: "Facing the Facts About Cancer."

A cover graphic asked, "Did you know: That cancer is NOT hereditary or contagious? That cancer is one of the most curable of all major causes of death? That there are only three accepted forms of cancer treatment?" Attention-grabbing, to be sure. Of course, we now know that in a small percentage of cases, cancer can be hereditary. The incorrect notion of contagion would sadly linger until the mid-1980s. With regard to cancer being curable (the goal at the time, although the term makes today's doctors shudder), early detection was indeed key. But for many reasons, perhaps as in Albert's case, fear left people frozen, unable to be more vigilant and insistent about an unusual symptom. As to the last question, those who were diagnosed were often so desperate for help, they were willing to try anything. The "three treatment" line was meant to dispel the myths spread by charlatans, who peddled salves, sweat boxes, needle injections, and "old Indian remedies."

The booklet's interior pages offered greater detail on the issues raised by the cover's questions. A disturbing graphic on page 27, however, was shockingly dramatic. It showed four hospital beds, topped by the heading "Of Every 4 Persons Who Have Cancer . . ." The caption below the first bed read, "One is saved by treatment . . . surgery, radium or x-ray" (the three treatments mentioned on the cover). Below the second bed was the text "One dies because cancer was discovered too late." The two last beds were linked together by a funeral wreath and the words "Two die in the absence of new discoveries." In other words, only 25 percent of those diagnosed in 1947 were expected to survive their disease. The cruel irony was that the information and graphics for this brochure had been provided by Mary and Albert Lasker.[8]

Three years later, when Albert was diagnosed, not much had changed in the way of treatment. Surgery could remove tumors, but in cases like his, where cancer had spread, the next line of defense was X-rays or radium. The latter was often injected directly into a tumor, though research into radioactivity had recently discovered that radioactive cobalt was even more effective than radium, and less costly. And while intriguing experiments were being done with mustard gas, a wartime chemical weapon, its application in cancer wouldn't be approved until later in the decade.

More troubling still was a newspaper article that had appeared three months before Albert's diagnosis. According to information coming from NCI, if cancer was found early, before spreading, the survival rate was 93 percent. NCI figures also showed that only 30 percent of cases were actually found early. The article went on, "If there is regional involvement, or beginning metastasis, the probability drops to 64%." The next line was not good news for the Laskers: "When cancer is found in several places in the body, the probability the patient will live a year or more drops to 29%."[9]

—

Dr. Sidney Farber graduated from Harvard Medical School in 1927 and became a resident pathologist at Children's Hospital in Boston. Farber studied the classifications of children's tumors and wrote a textbook on the subject. But treating actual patients was his passion. Sitting in his hospital basement lab one day, pondering treatment ideas, Farber determined to focus on one of cancer's saddest, and almost inevitably fatal, varieties: childhood lymphoblastic leukemia.

In 1947, Farber began a clinical trial using folic acid (or folate), a vitamin-like substance found in fruits and vegetables. Its crucial role in cell division spoke to him. The most rapidly dividing cells in the human body are blood cells. Perhaps, Farber postulated, folic acid could accelerate the rate of healthy blood cell division in leukemia patients, allowing the healthy cells to crowd out the diseased ones. However, the results were disastrously reversed: the folic acid increased the numbers of leukemic cells, not the healthy ones. He stopped the experiments immediately and struck on another theory. What if the reverse of folic acid would work? Thus the study of an anti-folate, a synthetic derivative of folic acid, began.[10]

Farber tested sixteen children who had been given up on as "hopeless" cases. Ten achieved temporary remission. The possibility of a new kind of cancer treatment was announced publicly on Friday, September 5, 1947. Called aminopterin, the "yellow powder" was received with enthusiasm by some in the field and with disbelief and resistance by others. The press grabbed on to it immediately. With the headline "Leukemia Victims' Life Span Prolonged," one April 9, 1948, article explained, "Dr. Sidney Farber said of 16 children treated since November 1947, 10 are living longer than the average time. One eight-year-old child was still living 20 months after diagnosis. Previously no child had survived longer than a year."[11]

This was indeed good news. But it was not the silver bullet everyone hoped for. More often than not, the improvement was only temporary, lasting just weeks to months. "The disease still smolders, flaring up again," Farber reported at an International Congress on Hematology. "It is not yet known why the drug produces temporary benefits in some cases, but not in others."[12]

But they were remissions nonetheless, previously unheard of in the deadly leukemia. Faber went on to publish a paper in the *New England Journal of Medicine* in June 1948. Writing about a bone marrow biopsy on a child who had been treated with aminopterin, he said, "The bone marrow looked so normal, that one could dream of a cure."[13]

Although Albert hadn't yet been diagnosed, there is little chance that such remarkable advances, coupled with the magic word "cure," would have escaped Mary's notice. She wanted to know more about the bright and creative mind of Sidney Farber, the first person who had found success with chemicals as therapy—chemotherapy. A letter to Mary from NCI director John Heller in September 1948 spoke encouragingly of just that: "This approach looks awfully good to me and we are tremendously interested in further exploration in the field. If longer and longer remissions can be achieved in some of these leukemias, not only is the patient more comfortable and hopeful but it allows more time for possible advances in chemotherapy along other lines. Definitely, I feel encouraged about this matter."[14]

Mary was encouraged, too. But when Albert was diagnosed two years later, and Mary learned it had spread to his lymph nodes, she knew he was in grave danger. His surgery might have made him "cancer-free," but she became desperately proactive. Through her contacts at NCI, she had met Dr. Freddy Homburger, a cancer researcher at Tufts College in Boston. She asked him if, for a fee, he would scour the country in person, interviewing anyone who might have some therapy they could use if Albert had a recurrence. Considering Farber's work and that of others, Mary also asked Homburger to be on the lookout for places she could lend financial support that might turn into clinical development.

Homburger's first stop was the basement lab of fellow Bostonian Sidney Farber. On a hunch, he asked Farber if he could test the increasingly successful aminopterin on colon cancer cells. Homburger's hypothesis was that if the drug was effective on one type of cancer, perhaps it could be useful on another type (a theory that has now proven to be true in some cases). Farber heartily agreed. But

Homburger's tests were unsuccessful, and after a number of other dead ends, he returned to Mary empty-handed.

～

Albert came home from the hospital in August. A few months later, in October, he wrote to his cousin in Israel relating stories about his surgeries and concluding, "The doctors tell me that if I am my own self within a year, I will have done well."[15] By this time, Albert had thoroughly regained his strength, and he bought a farm in Dutchess County, New York. It was near the town of Amenia, a hundred miles north of the city, near the Connecticut border. The 420 acres of rolling hills, fields, and forests is known by two names: Smithfield Farm and Heathcote. To the Laskers, it was simply "the farm." It came with a herd of Guernsey cows (just as Albert had had at Mill Road Farm) and a price tag of $150,000 ($1.7 million in 2023).

Work was begun immediately on a gardener's cottage and a guesthouse, while Mary undertook changes to the white Georgian main house. It had a stately presence, with front pillars and a lovely foyer. As she had at Beekman Place, she directed that nearly all the walls, carpets, and furniture were to be white. It would be the job of the artwork to add color. The Laskers had bought some new pieces and brought others from New York so that the farm would be just as elegant. And yet, it didn't feel like a cold museum. It was a house, according to a *McCall's* magazine spread, "where guests feel free to trail around in swimsuits and paper slippers, sit up half the night in bathrobes, talking, and get up when they feel like it. . . . Books and magazines are piled all over, and people are forever flopping down to read."[16]

When 1951 dawned, the Laskers' calendar might have been overwhelming if it hadn't been for the wonderful Jane McDonough. Just before they had left for Paris the year before, Mary had hired the lovely twenty-seven-year-old from Aberdeen, Mississippi, as her assistant. Smart and organized, Jane would help keep Mary's lobbying work in order, as well as the goings-on at the Lasker Foundation. It would be Jane who would help gather and categorize the ever-changing health statistics that Mary presented to members of Congress.

Jane would also help update the biennial Big Fact Book, and she was on the "notebook project." Some years earlier, Mary had gotten into the habit of using a four-inch-thick black notebook, using a new one for each month of the year. They were custom-made just for her, and she ordered them a dozen at a time. They served as diaries, address books, and datebooks, housing thousands of bits of information, and always containing a yard-long foldout page. The translucent onionskin was replete with the latest facts and figures that Mary used on her visits with scientists and members of Congress. She always had the current version at her fingertips around the house, and never left home without it stashed in her handbag.

Making certain productivity continued during Mary's frequent and lengthy trips to the beauty parlor each week was Jane's responsibility as well. They installed a private (and white) telephone in the salon so that Mary could place calls and so that incoming ones could be forwarded from Beekman Place. While Mary sat under the dryer, Jane took dictation of letters to be typed up back home. It wasn't long before she became Mary's close friend and confidant. Because they felt certain that all would be well under Jane's watchful eye, Mary and Albert kept up their whirlwind pace, heading to the La Quinta Hotel for their winter sojourn.

Their calendar overflowed: they hosted a luncheon in honor of actress and friend Greta Garbo, organized cocktails to celebrate author, editor, and publisher Bennett Cerf, and treated friends to dinner and dancing in La Quinta's Mirage Room. Only two events took Mary away from the March social flurry. The first was an ACS board meeting in Ohio (she had been on the board since its revamping four years before). From there she went back to New York for a few days, and then took a day trip to Washington for a meeting of the National Advisory Heart Council with Florence, followed by an appointment with President Truman. Newly divorced, Florence had purchased a house in Georgetown overlooking the Potomac. This would be the first time Mary would see the house. "I was determined to be where I had a view," Florence told her.

That day, Albert had heard about another van Gogh painting he coveted very much. *Roses* was stunning in its simplicity: white blooms in a green vase on a table, with traces of pale pink throughout the petals. It had actually been painted twice. The first one had a horizontal orientation; it belonged to statesman Averell Harriman. The second, vertically oriented, was one of twenty-seven paintings in Georg Hirschland's collection. A successful Jewish German banker, Hirschland had been increasingly harassed by the Nazi government and emigrated to the United States in 1937. However, his artwork had to remain behind, to be scooped up by the Nazis. Mary had found the story in an art book and shared it with Albert, who fell in love with both the saga and the painting.

Roses had been reconnected with Hirschland's heirs in 1950. It was now sequestered in a bank vault in New York, where a friend of Albert's learned it was for sale. Albert immediately called Mary from California, asking her to go see it. She explained that she was about to leave on the train for a meeting with the president and would go see the painting when she got back. He panicked, but she calmly assured him that her dealer instinct led her to believe it was safe; she assumed a painting locked away in a bank vault couldn't possibly rise to the consciousness of other collectors in a day.

When Mary returned to the city, she called the friend who had alerted Albert. To her horror, he told her she was too late. During the few hours she was in Washington, Georges Wildenstein, of Fifth Avenue's famous Wildenstein Gallery, had purchased the painting for $100,000. It had never occurred to Mary that a dealer might hear the same story Albert had. After a day of negotiations, and aided by Albert's son-in-law Leigh Block, Mary finally got Wildenstein to sell the glorious painting for $135,000. Mary's five-hour trip to Washington had cost Albert $7,000 an hour ($82,000 an hour today). But he wasn't angry with her. In fact, he related the story many times, always chuckling each time he told it.[17]

Back on the East Coast in April, the Laskers entertained lavishly and frequently both at Beekman Place and in Amenia. General Bill Donovan came for a visit, and Albert took him to see the farm. He told Albert, "Now you've become a real farmer." "Not a farmer," Albert replied. "I'm an agriculturist." Donovan asked him the difference. "A farmer," Albert explained," is one who makes money on the farm and loses it in the city. An agriculturist is one who makes money in the city and loses it on the farm."[18]

The Laskers headed to Europe for a few months in May 1951, stopping first in London for a stay with Mary's friend Audrey Pleydell-Bouverie. While Mary and Audrey had plenty to keep them entertained, Albert paid a call on seventy-six-year-old Winston Churchill. The former prime minister had been voted out of office in 1945, although he would return via another vote in October that year. Churchill had ample time to visit with Albert, and their cozy chat lasted four and a quarter hours.

At their eleven-year anniversary on June 21, it was apparent that Mary and Albert were not just husband and wife. They were friends and collaborators in everything, totally devoted to each other. "All she did," Albert explained, "was keep me from losing my mind."

~

Beauty surrounded the Laskers, and not just within their home. Both Mary and Albert loved flowers. As it had been with art, at the beginning Albert's love was visual, without the knowledge of what anything actually was. He had been enormously proud of the gardens at Mill Road Farm, even if he didn't know the name of a single plant. For Mary, however, that love was lifelong, as she had been well educated by her mother. Aside from Sara's personal gardens and the creation of the two city parks in Watertown, it was Sara who had instigated the terrace planting when she came to live with Mary after Frank died. And once she was established in New York, Sara became a member of the city's park association. Mary carried on that love after she and Albert moved to Beekman Place; fresh flowers graced every room every day.

It had troubled Mary, though, that the New York City streets she traveled on were so plain and dirty. So in 1942, a plan to spruce up Manhattan had sprouted in her head. After Albert sold Mill Road Farm to the University of Chicago, the head of the university's botany department began experimenting with chrysanthemums on the property, eventually creating a winter-hardy variety. Mary bought up two million seeds and presented them to the New York City parks commissioner in honor of her mother. Covering the cost for their planting in Central Park, she named the beautiful garden the Sara Woodard Memorial Chrysanthemum Plantings.

The next spring, the city harvested seeds from that first bloom, and Mary, along with Alice, went on a letter-writing campaign as "crusaders"—the term Alice used when quoted in a newspaper story. They offered free seeds to colleges, parks, hospitals, housing authorities, and garden clubs across America and beyond, ultimately sending off half a million seeds. Queen Elizabeth even received some and planted them at Windsor Castle. Albert was bemused, thinking it was a rather eccentric idea. But those chrysanthemums made a spectacular display of color during the fall right through November, long after all other blooms were gone.

Driving on Park Avenue some years later, Mary felt that the avenue's center malls were unbearably dull. Tulips would do the trick, she thought. In 1949, she donated enough bulbs for four blocks of Park Avenue median below Grand Central Station. The city's garden experts said tulips could never live there; smoke, soot, and car exhaust would kill them. "Well," Mary later explained, "I said that I'd like to do a test planting anyway, and would they mind if I gave them the money to do this." The city gave way, telling her she could waste her money any way she wanted to. The tulips came up beautifully the next spring, and every spring after that, making another splendid burst of color. Mary had a new cause.

About the time the Central Park chrysanthemums were in full bloom in 1951, four Lasker Awards were presented at Midtown Manhattan's Roosevelt Hotel. This brought the total to twenty-seven since their inception. Mary and Albert realized that not only were their awards helping the recipients financially, they were bringing the little-known researchers publicity as well. Receiving the Lasker Award frequently led to other honors. Carl Ferdinand Cori, a 1946 recipient, had won a Nobel Prize in 1947, and more would go on to do so. While the work of all twenty-seven awardees was important, Mary's dream of a cure for cancer still had not materialized. As if sensing an approaching enemy, the disease remained elusive and mercilessly deadly.

—

In January 1952, Albert's abdominal distress returned. As far as Mary knew, he was still unaware that he had cancer. He made the trip back up to Columbia-Presbyterian at 168th Street for a routine checkup, which extended over three days. When the checkup was completed, Albert was sent back home, miraculously feeling fine. But in February the pain returned, this time much sharper, though he felt well enough to have a small dinner party the night before checking in on the seventeenth. The cancer had returned, doctors explained to Mary, and there was nothing more to be done. Albert was told he had a liver problem that would necessitate prolonged treatment. If he suspected cancer, he kept it to himself. Mary moved into a room in the Harkness Pavilion next to his, but that was the only concession he would allow. He insisted she continue living as normally as possible until he came home.

News reports of his hospitalization were jolly, not unlike Albert's demeanor itself: "Albert D. Lasker who's being checked up on at the Harkness Pavilion, appears to be in good health (and wealth too)."[19] A month later, the papers extolled the recognition and awards Mary had received from ACS and the American Heart Association. Later in the month, they wrote about Mary having dinner with Florence, U.S. Senate secretary Leslie Biffle, and Vice President Alben Barkley and his wife, followed by going to see the Broadway production of *Guys and Dolls*.

Meanwhile, Albert continued to hold court in the Harkness Pavilion, welcoming business associates, family members, and friends, including President Truman's daughter, Margaret, and Eleanor Roosevelt. He even bought two paintings from his hospital bed, one by Henri Fantin-Latour and a small Picasso. He gossiped with friends and discussed world affairs. Greta Garbo sent him freshly squeezed California orange juice, and artist friends Salvador Dalí and Henri Matisse hand-painted get-well cards.

Equally important was the news that a wing of Memorial Hospital had designated forty-two beds as a chemotherapy wing. The Laskers had donated funds to provide "ten fellowships which will enable the city-run hospital to be staffed by outstanding men and women in this field." Some chemicals, an article explained, "have brought comfort and longer life to patients whose types of cancer respond neither to knife or ray. A distant beacon has been illuminated."

It was the beacon Mary had been hoping and praying for. Unbeknownst to Albert, she was still working frantically, almost maniacally, from her Harkness room. She called everyone she had ever met who had a connection to cancer research. In addition to asking what they might be working on that could be administered to her husband, she asked for referrals to other researchers. Money was no object—but time certainly was.

The Laskers kept an eye on Washington as well. In early May, Congress voted more money for NIH. As Mary explained it, "The additional increases totaled about $5,300,000, which was really very small. This money was divided roughly between the cancer and heart institutes. The heart institute received an additional $700,000 for intramural research [research within NIH] and about $800,000 more than it would have otherwise received for project grants-in-aid." (Grants-in-aid come from the government for a specific project.) She continued, "The Cancer Institute's grants-in-aid project was increased . . . , and its intramural research about half a million." Even if it wasn't anywhere near what they had hoped for, Mary said it was still worth having made the effort, and not just for the institutes. It made Albert happy when she shared the phone calls and newspaper stories.

Then, slowly, cancer took its toll. Albert and Mary's love for each other was never more pronounced than in those last days. He slipped into a coma, and at 8:00 a.m. on May 30, 1952, Albert Lasker died. Mary's first call was to Jane, saying, "He slipped away from me."[20]

Chapter 7

~

"We Did It the Hard Way"

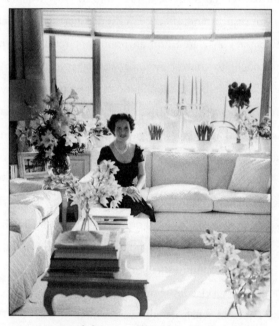

Mary in the living room of her Beekman Place home, circa 1960s.

66 I never felt so helpless in my life. I knew he was dying, and there was
nothing I could do to help him," Mary remembered. "I thought of all
we had done together to fight cancer, and this—his death—was our
reward. I felt completely defeated."[1]

Mary held a small, private funeral for Albert on June 1, and then made
plans for his interment. Alice's architect husband, Al Fordyce, designed a beautiful private mausoleum to be placed in a parklike setting within Sleepy Hollow

Cemetery in Westchester County, New York. In the company of other industry titans' graves—including Walter Chrysler, Andrew Carnegie, and William A. Rockefeller Jr. (John D.'s brother and co-founder of Standard Oil)—the white marble structure was elegant in its simplicity, with twin lead-paned windows facing each other that brought in the sunlight. "It was such a pretty landscape," Mary said, "a beautiful scene with a little brook running through. Albert would have liked it."

He was eulogized in both the House and the Senate. And in addition to widespread obituary coverage, Albert was lionized with wonderful anecdotes, written with pure respect and affection. Given Albert's time spent in Florida, the *Tallahassee Democrat* considered him an important resident, writing, "One of the diseases he sought to control by underwriting research into its cause and cure ironically killed him, but the foundation he laid may one day end the fatal toll and the dread of cancer."[2] The *Wisconsin Jewish Chronicle* recognized his philanthropy: "Man of wealth and ability, he gave of both unsparingly in the advancement of human betterment. As such, he will be long remembered and sorely missed."[3] His friend Leonard Lyon, a syndicated columnist, wrote an eloquent tribute, ending with: "There should be no groping for the name when the deeds of Albert Lasker are recounted. Our nation is the greater for his having lived."[4]

Watching a person in their final moments, wondering if each breath will be their last, is an emotionally exhausting event. So is making phone calls to loved ones, planning a service (even a simple one), and, in Mary's case, dealing with the press. The void when it's all over, combined with grief and sadness, is a dark, lonely place. Mary was very adept at compartmentalizing her emotions. If she visited that dark place, she did so privately. Her anger, however, was public.

"I was more determined than ever to obtain more funds for research against cancer and heart and other major killers and cripplers of our time," she recalled. "I realized even more pointedly how little was known." Those killers had robbed Mary of people she loved. Her drive to cure them was now a quest of such magnitude, it could only be described as a *crusade*. There would be no more excuses; no one and nothing would stand in her way.

At the end of June, Mary made her first trip to Washington after Albert's death. She attended a meeting of the National Advisory Heart Council, and then two days later, on a Sunday afternoon, she and Florence went to visit President Truman. He had chosen not to run for another term in the upcoming November election, but he could still have an impact in terms of the NIH budget.

The women suggested it would be a wonderful legacy if the president made certain that adequate funds were available for the institutes established during his administration. They had consulted with those institute heads, they told him, as well as others, to ascertain the sums that could be used effectively in the coming year. The specifics they presented were $25 million for cancer, $37 million for heart disease, $27 million for mental health, $18 million for arthritis and metabolic diseases, and $15 million for neurological diseases and blindness. The total was a whopping $122 million. Would the president write a letter to Frederick Lawton, the budget director, asking for their figures?

Truman stood up and smiled. "You'll see. There will be an improvement."

The next morning, the two thought of another avenue to further support Truman's promise. Mary telephoned Wallace Graham, the president's personal physician, to ask him to remind the president of their important visit. His response was completely unexpected. "Well, you've given me a fine job, haven't you?" he told Mary. She was confused. "The president," he went on, "has dumped all that stuff you brought him yesterday on my desk, and I'm to take up the matter with the budget boys. I'm not such a good one to do this; I've already gotten after them too much on things I'm interested in." It appeared the future of NIH funding now rested in a rather unwilling physician's hands.

Graham wanted to know whom else he might be able to speak with about their proposed figures. They suggested Dr. Scheele, the surgeon general, as the perfect choice. There wasn't much more they could do, and Mary left for Europe in July. The Continent held good memories that she was certain would recharge her.

When she returned in September, she and Florence again met with the president, asking what had been decided between him and the budget office regarding additional NIH funding. As they learned repeatedly, no matter how friendly the man who sat behind the desk in the Oval Office, his focus seemed to always be hampered by the principle "out of sight, out of mind." In an effort to redeem himself, Truman called his secretary, Matt Connolly, and asked whether a budget letter had been sent. Connolly was unsure, and the meeting ended. Mary's heart sank. She called Dr. Graham again, who promised to look into it. But after weeks of leaving him additional unanswered phone messages, Mary and Florence needed a new approach. The last time the budget letter had been seen was in Connolly's office, so that's where they went.

"Well, you know," Connolly told them, "the only one who can get anything done if she really wants to is Mrs. Truman." Why hadn't he told them that before? Florence knew Bess Truman fairly well, and called her that afternoon. The First Lady, charming and powerful as she was, had seldom used her influence. But budget increases to spare Americans from suffering appealed to her as a last important step she and the president could take before leaving Washington. Mrs. Truman did, indeed, talk to the president, who again took the matter up with Connolly. Within a week, the president had written a memo stating in no uncertain terms that the additional funds requested for NIH be added to the budget.

Speaking of their relentless campaigning for medical research, President Truman once joked with Anna that Mary and Florence were the worst lobbyists he had ever known. But privately, to his family, he acknowledged that, in truth, they "were the most tireless, consistent, and effective crusaders he had ever known."[5]

Indeed they were. As Mary later observed, "Powerful men could have gotten the job done much faster. . . . We did it the hard way."

⁓

A clause in the original Articles of Confederation states: "No Money shall be drawn from the Treasury, but in Consequence of Appropriations made by Law; and a regular Statement and Account of Receipts and Expenditures of all public Money shall be published from time to time."[6]

Thus was born the mysterious appropriations process. However, while the Constitution grants Congress the power to fund the federal government, it doesn't specify the exact budgeting process Congress is to follow. By the time Mary and Florence learned the difference between approval and appropriation in 1944, the government's financial responsibility had grown far beyond what the Founding Fathers had envisaged. And those good gentlemen could never have imagined the convoluted chain of events that appropriations had become.

The process begins at the end of each fiscal year, when the executive branch (including the president, the cabinet, and the budget office—in Truman's time the Bureau of the Budget, now the Office of Management and Budget) develops a proposed budget for the next fiscal year and submits it to the legislative branch. Then, traveling a path similar to the steel ball in a pinball machine, the budget pings between the Senate and House, which draw up bills to fund it. The president may either sign those bills or reject them and send them back to Congress for further discussions. This cycle continues until everyone agrees.

The House and Senate Appropriations Committees have a number of subcommittees, each of which is responsible for funding a different area. The chairs of those appropriations subcommittees align with whatever political party enjoys the majority. Once Mary and Florence understood the appropriations process, it didn't take long for them to figure out that those men (they were *all* men in this era) were powerful indeed and the ones to make friends with. Furthermore, they learned that while Republicans and Democrats differed on many counts, they worked in a surprisingly collegial atmosphere. That was particularly true when it came to issues of health—cancer and heart disease don't select targets based on political leanings. Members of one party sometimes even mentored members of the opposing party. Such was the case of John Fogarty.

A Rhode Island Democrat, Fogarty arrived in the House of Representatives in 1941 and was assigned to the Appropriations Committee six years later. He was hoping for a position on the Defense Department appropriations subcommittee but was assigned instead to the Labor-FSA subcommittee, which was charged with financing the Labor Department and the Federal Security Agency. Fogarty was initially disappointed—and bored. But that slowly changed as he watched the Wisconsin Republican who chaired the subcommittee. Congressman Frank Keefe was zealous about improving the nation's health and believed that the government's investment in it, and medical research, needed increasing. Little would get done, he said, if researchers were just "fiddling along" with modest annual budget increases. This attitude, and the fact he was from Wisconsin, brought Keefe to Mary's attention again. She and Florence had visited him in 1948, and as a consequence he became immensely instrumental in shepherding through funding increases for the various institutes.[7]

Fogarty's passion for America's health took root and blossomed profusely under Keefe's tutelage. And that came to Mary's attention as well. While the mentor and mentee developed a friendship, Mary began to make frequent visits to Fogarty's office. When the Democrats took back the House in 1948, Fogarty became the subcommittee chair. As the ranking member, Keefe's influence continued until his retirement in 1951. In a letter to his Republican mentor that same year, Fogarty wrote. "I'd like to extend to you once more my own heartfelt thanks for the help which you gave me, without which I should have been unable to advance along the course charted by you years ago."[8]

It was Fogarty who had gotten the NIH increases just before Albert's death, along with his Democratic counterpart in the Senate, Dennis Chavez of New Mexico. Fogarty was in top form again a year later, in May 1953, defending increased appropriations. As Mary remembered, "He did a stirring and superb job supporting additional funds for hospital construction and for rehabilitation, and various other items." More remarkable, Fogarty had managed to convince fellow representatives that research was necessary even in the face of the ongoing Korean War.

But Fogarty's spirited rhetoric about the need for greater research—including for heart disease—contributed to a horrible irony. Two weeks later, John Fogarty suffered a heart attack that would take him back to Rhode Island for a three-month recuperation. It was a reminder of the fragility of life, and of the importance of his voice in Mary's crusade.

~

The American Medical Association had originally been caught off guard when President Truman first mentioned nationalized health insurance in 1945. That was the last time they were unprepared. Soon after the first health message, every AMA member was assessed $25, resulting in a war chest of $2.5 million. Then, taking a page out of Albert Lasker's manual on how to sway public opinion, they hired the high-powered public relations firm Whitaker and Baxter in San Francisco. The firm launched a campaign against national health insurance, with a focus on the failures of the British health plan.[9] The message suggested that government interference would result in a loss of freedom when it came to scientific research, and that the ability of the investigator, not the money, was what counted most in scientific progress. Also creeping in was an egotistical notion that the opinions of laypeople (in other words, government officials and citizen lobbyists) were driven by emotion and not the knowledge gained in medical schools.

The AMA took aim at Senator Claude Pepper as well. A campaign dubbing him "Red Pepper" (intended not as a comment on his red hair but to smear his progressive views as socialist or Communist) caused him to be defeated in his 1950 bid for reelection. Mary lost a powerful Senate ally. When General Dwight D. Eisenhower swept in as the new president in 1952, defeating the Democratic candidate Adlai Stevenson in a landslide, her crusade lost an ally in the White House as well.

Mary was vexed by Americans' perception of illness. Diagnoses of heart disease and cancer were nearly always sentences to a life of disability or, worse, death. Since there was little to be done, people took the proverbial ostrich approach and simply ignored ill health. Those beliefs also kept citizens from applying pressure on their representatives in Washington to support the advancement of research. That made politicians' work less complicated, to be sure. It was easy to rally citizen support for defense against a Communist attack—a common fear, albeit a rather unlikely possibility. But it was far more difficult to rally the same support for defense against deadly diseases. And, according to the facts and figures in Mary's omnipresent black notebook, becoming seriously ill was a real possibility for most Americans over the course of their lifetime.

When she was successful, Mary found her work fulfilling. The rest of the time it felt like a tremendous weight she was forever dragging uphill. But around this time a spectacular distraction captured Mary's attention: the coronation of the young British queen. "It was something that would give me special pleasure, and one not likely to be repeated in my lifetime," Mary remembered.

Twenty-seven-year-old Elizabeth Alexandra Mary Windsor had become queen immediately upon the death of her father, just a few weeks before Albert's death in 1952. But in the tradition of respect, her coronation festivities—a nine-hundred-year-old Westminster Abbey tradition—were delayed until Tuesday, June 2, 1953. After a comfortable four-day first-class voyage aboard the *Queen Elizabeth*, Mary would be just one of a predicted one million tourists who would pour into London for the event. But she wouldn't have to put up in a hotel, again staying in the beautiful home of Audrey Pleydell-Bouverie.

When dawn broke on coronation day, the weather was a disappointment: rain, chilly winds, and the threat of thunder and hail. But the celebratory spirit of the city was not to be dampened. The Westminster Abbey ceremony began at eleven o'clock in the morning, with the crown of glittering jewels placed on the queen's head at twelve-thirty.[10] Mary wasn't at the actual crowning; even her money couldn't garner that ticket. But an hour later, when the queen climbed into her golden carriage for a five-mile procession through the heart of London, Mary was waiting as a guest at Apsley House on Piccadilly, at the corner of Hyde Park. The former mansion of the Duke of Wellington was now a museum, and the only thing left on that part of the street that had not been destroyed during the Blitz. So when the queen, resplendent in a bejeweled white satin gown, rode slowly past, Mary and the others on the Apsley House balconies were the only people for her to wave to. It was tremendously exciting.

That night, in a pink lace Dior ball gown, Mary joined the celebration at the swankiest of the coronation parties, dubbed the "ball of the century." The entire first floor of the Savoy Hotel had been turned into a veritable fantasia. More than fourteen hundred guests paid $35 ($375 today) for the charity soirée, and were treated to dinner, dancing, and Maurice Chevalier's floor show. The queen's sister, Princess Margaret, joined other members of the nobility at the ball, although the queen and her husband, Prince Philip, did not attend. The partiers drank three thousand bottles of champagne and capped off the night watching a massive fireworks show, which ended just before dawn.[11]

It was all magnificent. However, it brought into focus the sharp contrast between a glittering life of privilege and wealth and one of poverty, disease, and disability. Mary had actually had a guilty conscience about even going to England. The Senate Appropriations Committee had not yet met, and she felt they had a real chance to raise the NIH budget figures, given that there were a number of senators who were in favor of the idea. The urge to do one more round of meetings with them overtook her, and she booked an early return back to New York on June 12.

While the congressional debates and votes were exciting, they were just a small part of the days Mary spent in Washington. More often, she and Florence would bounce between the office buildings of the Senate and House, weaving up and down the corridors to meet with decision-makers. Sometimes they had to wait for an hour or more if an official was tied up in another meeting. Everyone they saw received a copy of the most recent fact sheet, enumerating diagnoses, deaths, and dollars. Trips to NIH headquarters in Bethesda, Maryland, figured in as well, where they gathered data from NIH officials and courted any who were—amazingly—still skeptical of government funding for their research.

Even Mary's train travel between New York and Washington was productive. Leaving in the early afternoon from Grand Central Station, her private compartment was equipped with a telephone, and was soon cluttered with reports and articles. When she arrived at Washington's Union Station four hours later, she would have just enough time to change for cocktails and dinner, almost always for the purpose of discussing upcoming legislation, discoveries, or testimony. The return trip was an afternoon journey, too, spent exactly as the outbound travel had been.

These trips had been far less stressful during the Truman administration than they were under the new administration of President Eisenhower. Early on, Mary and Florence had hoped that one of his appointees would be particularly helpful. Oveta Culp Hobby had been appointed head of the Federal Security

Agency, but she had her eye on a cabinet position. The president had campaigned on the idea of creating a Department of Health, Education and Welfare (HEW), which would suit Hobby just fine. But that department's birth would depend on the AMA—if not their support, at least not their opposition. And Hobby knew it.

Mary and Florence invited her to dinner. "She came very prettily dressed," Mary described, "amiable, noncommittal, sympathetic, but cautious." Hobby didn't know much about her dinner hostesses, just that they were generally interested in medical research. The citizen lobbyists hoped their shared gender would sway Hobby's thoughts about budget increases for research. But once they saw past Hobby's pleasant demeanor, they realized that no help would be forthcoming. She needed the AMA; if it was against federal research funding, she had to take the same position. HEW was indeed created and Hobby was named its first director, becoming only the second woman to serve in the cabinet. She remained loyal to the AMA's positions, and pleasant but cool toward Mary and Florence's crusade.

Their frustrations didn't end there. The atmosphere of the Eisenhower administration was one of opposition to anything that had been done under Truman. That included the budget. They'd have to find other inroads.

⁓

In Albert's absence, most of Mary's waking hours were dedicated to her work. When she awoke each day at midmorning (she required nine hours of sleep, which truly irked her), she had breakfast in bed. Along with her sliced oranges, cottage cheese, and coffee, she read newspapers and scanned her mail. Then, still in bed, Mary began her daily phone calls. She fully admitted to being addicted to telephones, acknowledging that while Albert had had no problem lavishing her with jewels and furs, he insisted she pay her own phone bills.

By one o'clock, Mary was dressed and headed out for lunch, typically some kind of business meeting, followed by another meeting in midafternoon. After a return home for a change of clothing, there would be one or two cocktail dates and then dinner (again, mostly business). Her few social dinners were typically for six or eight, and followed by the opera or theater. Mary's schedule varied only if she had a morning meeting. Large parties at her home—those with 80 to 150 guests—served a purpose. Ideas, Mary realized early on, typically don't come out of thin air. They arose from people talking to one another. As time went on, she would refine the choreography of putting together the right mix.[12]

Wealthy people are sometimes parsimonious, a possible reason for their wealth. Albert had enjoyed his money; he loved earning it and he loved giving it away. But he had told Mary that it was useless to go to friends to raise money. They'll then ask for support of their causes, and, as Mary explained, "you are constantly in a position of exchanging money with friends." Mary had adopted many of Albert's financial beliefs, particularly his advice to go to the government for big research dollars. That was paying off, but there were still reasons to give her own money.

When it came to campaign contributions, Mary was very calculating. An acquaintance once said, "The Laskers don't *buy* votes. They *reward* votes."[13] As she had when Albert was alive, Mary gave modest contributions meant to show appreciation and encouragement for a continuing upward movement in research funding. Her sister, Alice, later explained, "People don't understand that Mary gives money as men or corporations give it—professionally, not emotionally."[14] In that regard, Mary was not partisan. She made contributions to Republicans Keefe and Bridges just as she gave to Democrats Pepper and Fogarty.

Mary also didn't scatter money around, which prevented doing "big good," as Anna described. People who do that, Anna continued, "are too busy doing 'little good' in too many directions. Mary has always known exactly what she wants and won't be sidetracked."[15] Sometimes Mary's checks found their way directly to NCI, NIH, or one of the other institutes, but that, too, was calculated, as she became familiar with specific researchers and their projects.

One of Albert's greatest lessons was the importance of publicity, including well-written and well-placed articles and speeches. In these cases, Mary deferred to professionals, hiring a lobbyist—"a rather inadequate lobbyist," in her words—early on when she and Florence began working toward the creation of NIMH. His job during his tenure was to arrange for hearings and witnesses to increase funds for the institute. However, his work wasn't of the caliber that Mary was hoping for. The mental health connection, however, led her to a man who became her superstar.

⟋

Thomas Francis Xavier Gorman was the epitome of a New York Irishman. Nicknamed "Mike," he was irreverent, brash, and egotistical. Feisty from the top of his red-haired head to the toes of his always polished oxfords, he possessed all the qualities necessary to be effective in Washington. Gorman enlisted in the army at the outset of World War II and spent four years overseas, writing feature articles, copy for news services, camp newspapers, and Air Corps radio shows. His last assignment was at Tinker Field, near Oklahoma City, and he chose to stay in the state after being discharged from the service, getting a job at the *Daily Oklahoman.* By chance, one day he was assigned a lead about the conditions at the state psychiatric institution, Central State Hospital.[16]

What Gorman found sickened and appalled him: filthy conditions, patient neglect, staff shortages. His journalistic mind led him to investigate other state hospitals, where he found similar conditions, all the result of funding shortages. The series of articles he wrote about these "snake pits" created public outrage, and that, in turn, gave birth to a grassroots campaign to reform Oklahoma's mental health care system. A condensed version of his articles appeared in the September 1948 *Reader's Digest.* And that's when he came to Florence's attention.

Waiting for an appointment one day, she randomly picked up that issue of *Reader's Digest.* She was thoroughly impressed with his research and writing, and thought a similar series might be good for the *Miami Daily News.* As they had in Oklahoma, the Miami articles received phenomenal response.

Mary saw the *Reader's Digest* article, too. She was so moved, she made certain Gorman was recognized by the Lasker Foundation, receiving the Award for Public Service the same year. Mary liked him and hired him frequently on a freelance basis for the citizen lobbyists' work.[17]

Gorman came to the attention of the AMA as well—or, rather, the attention of their PR firm. Whitaker and Baxter had originally tapped him to write their 1948 hit piece about the failures of the British health care system. Their offer of a free trip to England hadn't impressed him; he'd been there during the war. The mission didn't impress him either, given what he had seen with the lack of funding in the mental health arena. So Gorman (persuaded by Mary) took a temporary job with the Democratic National Committee and wrote a press release entitled "Lobbying Against Human Needs." The AMA, he wrote, was the "best financed lobby" in the country. But not a penny of the money it raised "went to medical research, scholarship for qualified would-be doctors or nurses, or the furthering of scientific programs to end needless suffering"—the very things one might have thought the AMA should focus on.

Mary also hired Gorman to freelance for her Committee for the Nation's Health, as well as for the National Committee Against Mental Illness (which would later become the National Committee on Mental Health). When their previous lobbyist—who had also served as the committee's executive secretary— was finally sent packing, Gorman stepped into the position. His job was broader, given his talents: take a bird's-eye view of the entire medical research landscape, along with greasing the lobbying wheels.

He was highly effective in prepping the citizen witnesses Mary selected, who were crucial to the legislative hearings. He had to significantly coach some of them, particularly physicians fond of using technical terms: "I *forbid* doctors to use the term 'myocardial infarction.' I say, 'You call it a heart attack or you leave the room.'"[18]

To be successful at anything in Washington, one must be driven, clever, and thick-skinned. Mary was certainly all of those things, and while some loved her for it, there were those who did not. She was criticized as being imperious, her facts and figures overwhelming. Gorman became very adept at smoothing the feathers she might have ruffled, plying legislators with alcohol and stroking their egos. And while Florence's calm approach might have suited some, she wasn't good with numbers and didn't use statistics in support of her positions. That left some politicians wondering why she'd come to their office and what they'd just been asked to do. Gorman followed up with those legislators, too, providing documents to clarify the points Florence had made during her visit. Together, the dynamic duo became the tenacious troika, and a well-orchestrated machine.

In July 1955, Senate majority leader (and Mary's new friend) Lyndon Johnson suffered a major heart attack. The forty-six-year-old was described as "seriously ill." Two months later, President Eisenhower was also struck by a heart attack, although his was listed as "mild." Those two pieces of news might well have brought to Americans' minds the notion that, no matter how powerful, famous, or wealthy someone is, they're still a human being, still susceptible to the same conditions as the powerless, unknown, and poor. Americans might also have begun wondering when, if ever, scientists would find ways to prevent the number one killer in the country.

When the Democrats took back both the House and Senate in November, Mary's work became somewhat easier. John Fogarty was a mighty force in the House, and now Lister Hill, an Alabama Democrat, was filling a similar role in the Senate. When Chavez decided to move from chairing the health appropriations subcommittee to its defense counterpart, Hill succeeded him, thanks to Florence's persuasive powers. He would ultimately be dubbed "Mr. Health" in the Senate. But there was a great deal of work to be done first.[19]

As had been true during Eisenhower's first term, the president's love-hate relationship with medical research continued in his second term, commencing in 1957. On the one hand, Eisenhower wanted to encourage the "people programs," those that erased the notion that conservatives were miserly and uncaring in the face of dying Americans. On the other hand, he was attentive to fellow conservatives who whispered in his ear that research was being pushed too fast. It was a struggle between hitting the gas pedal and pumping the brakes.

Sitting on Ike's desk in late summer 1960 was one of the last appropriations bills he would review as president. Congress had already approved the $547 million in it for NIH. That amount was $147 million more than the president had asked for, and he was inclined to veto it. With no friends in the White House to sway his opinion, Mary dove deep into her book of supporters and devised a plan.

The president loved his golf game and frequently played with a good friend of Jules Stein's. Stein was president of the Music Corporation of America, and a good friend of Mary's. She persuaded Stein to persuade the president's golf partner to impress upon the chief executive what might happen to Americans if he vetoed the NIH money.

To further make the point, Mary flew Dr. Sidney Farber from Boston to the golf game—which was being played in Newport, Rhode Island—to paint the picture of the two possible futures, depending on what the president did. Farber put the scenario in terms to which the president could relate. When Eisenhower had led the Allies in the D-Day invasion, it was successful because every available weapon and resource was at his disposal. That was what was being asked for now, in the battle against a disease as feared as the Nazis.

The president saw the light. He directed an aide to call the HEW secretary and make an appointment with him for Farber. The doctor was authorized to inform the secretary that the president was 100 percent behind the proposed NIH budget. And there would be no veto.[20]

⤳

"Every civilized city in the world—London, Rome, Paris—has trees and flowers. Americans flock to European cities. We could get more visitors if New York was as beautiful as it could be." Mary drove this point home to New York mayor Robert Wagner and his parks commission. Who were they to argue? Mary had already done more than anyone else to beautify Manhattan. After the Central Park tribute to Sara and the tulip planting in the median of Park Avenue for four blocks below Grand Central Station, Mary decided flowers should be everywhere the people were.

First, she and her stepchildren oversaw the planting of 180 flowering cherry trees, in Albert's honor, on the north side of the newly constructed United Nations building. Beneath the trees, more than forty thousand white daffodils would bloom every spring. Mary's next target was twenty-two blocks of the Park Avenue median above Grand Central. Here, she directed that alternating blocks of tulips and white daffodils were to be planted. As before, the city argued that the flowers wouldn't live, and as before, they were wrong. The 150,000-flower display was so spectacular that a taxi driver screeched his cab to a halt, sniffed the air, and proclaimed, "It even smells good!" The final stamp of approval of

Mary's plan came from the haughty *New Yorker* magazine, which wrote, "God bless Mary Lasker!"

The city was warming to the idea of flowers, and in 1957 it committed $309,500 for plantings where Mary's magic wand hadn't already landed. By the time her "Salute to Seasons" idea was launched at a Waldorf-Astoria luncheon, the flower fan club had grown considerably. Along with Anna, she reminded New Yorkers that half a million tourists flocked to Washington, D.C., every spring just to see cherry blossoms. Tourism equaled money, and that fact got the attention of businessmen, who had previously only thought of flowers on Mother's Day. Mary employed the same tactics in her beautification quest as she did with medical research: put up a little seed money, create a committee, and then sit back to watch it all bloom.

By 1960, the Salute to Seasons included elaborate lighting, paid for by a real estate corporation, that turned the cavernous dark streets into a "fairyland," according to one newspaper. Manhattan banks climbed on board, financing the planting of entire blocks of city streets. Changes of the seasons were acknowledged not only with flowers and decorations but with special entertainment as well. Patriotic songs rang out to celebrate the Fourth of July, and Christmas carols filled the frosty December days.[21]

City beautification and medical research might seem unrelated. Mary saw them as branches of the same family tree. "Urban renewers don't seem to realize that people need space for trees and shrubs. They need flowers in the spring and berries in the fall. It reassures them." She knew firsthand that being surrounded by beautiful things lifted the spirit. Not everyone could afford a grand house and original artwork. Plants did the same thing at a fraction of the price. They were comforting, too, as she explained. "Flowers are just little things to keep me from being depressed until a cure is found for diseases."

Chapter 8

~

"We Thought We'd Have More Time"

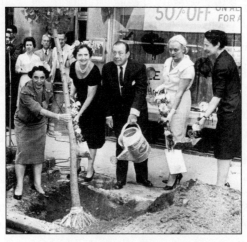

*Mary and Anna Rosenberg Hoffman planting a tree with
New York mayor Robert Wagner, early 1960s.*

T he very young-looking—and very skinny—senator from Massachusetts seemed an unlikely candidate for president. His arms were too
long for his coat and his pants weren't right at the bottom. Were they
rolled up? Nonetheless, Mary had one very positive memory of that first meeting with John Fitzgerald Kennedy: "He had a wonderful smile." He would soon
win her over, along with much of America.

Kennedy—Jack to friends and family—was the son of former ambassador
Joe Kennedy. Mary knew Joe, but she knew his wife, Rose, better. And she had

heard a great deal about Jack from Florence. Since the Kennedys maintained a home in Palm Beach and had long been celebrities among the Florida Democrats, they became friends of the Mahoneys. Jack had been a champion swimmer at Harvard, a World War II hero, and an author. The finishing touch to his presidential image was his beautiful wife, Jacqueline (Jackie) Bouvier.

Florence's affection for Kennedy influenced Mary to get to know him better. The young senator always stopped to chat with her when they passed in the halls of the Capitol. And when she hosted a dinner-dance at the members-only F Street Club in late 1959, Kennedy popped in for a couple of quick drinks and dances. A few weeks later, Florence invited Mary and the Kennedys over for dinner. She wanted to give Mary the opportunity to get to know them better, but Kennedy had an ulterior motive, and her name was Eleanor Roosevelt.

"Now why is she so much against me?" Kennedy asked Mary, apparently assuming, since both she and Eleanor lived in New York, they must be friends.

"Well, I really don't know what her attitude is," Mary told him. "But I know one thing: she's a person who is very fair. And the thing for you to do is go see her and ask her. Whatever she has to say, or to criticize about you, she'll tell you, and you'll be able to clear it up."

Kennedy did call on the former First Lady, and she was very up-front with him, as Mary had promised. Her concern was the same as that of many others in the Democratic Party: he was a Catholic. No Catholic had ever been president, and he would have an uphill battle facing a likely non-Catholic Republican. Rightly or wrongly, the notion being passed around was that Kennedy would put his faith—and by extension, the pope—ahead of his duties as chief executive. Ergo, the pope would be running America.

However, on Saturday, January 2, 1960, forty-two-year-old Jack Kennedy officially announced his candidacy for president of the United States. He was confident, he said, he would "win both the nomination and the election."[1] He campaigned deftly, fanning out his wife, parents, brothers, and sisters to help him cover every inch of the country. When the Democratic convention opened in the Los Angeles Coliseum on July 11, Kennedy would have six main competitors, including Senate majority leader Lyndon Johnson of Texas and former Illinois governor Adlai Stevenson.

Mary knew all of the candidates, but she knew Stevenson the best, having first met him during his 1952 presidential run. After a campaign rally that year, she and Florence were waiting for him at his private train car. "Here's a contribution for you," Mary had told him, check in hand, "but there are strings attached."

"I suppose they're ropes!" Stevenson had replied. "What are they?"

"Well, if you're elected, I expect half an hour of your time," Mary threw back at him, "and if you're not, I expect a great deal more." She was, of course, speaking in terms of her research lobbying, but a friendship was born.

As time passed, Stevenson became Mary's frequent escort, whether in New York, Chicago, or Europe. When rumors about a potential marriage circulated, Stevenson denied them. A newspaper writer pointed out, however, he kept denying he was running for president again, too.[2] And there he was, being considered for the Democratic nomination for a third time. This put Mary in a quandary. As a friend, she felt she should be for him, although Stevenson was not even for himself, she would later say. She didn't think he could succeed in such a crowded and charismatic field. But she again donated to his campaign, shared some publicity ideas with him, and covered the costs of his newspaper ads.

A week before the convention, Mary arrived in Los Angeles with Florence in tow. They stayed at the lush Beverly Hills Hotel and hopped from one Stevenson event to another: rallies, dinners, and even a massive breakfast the morning the convention began. As Mary settled into her seat in the Coliseum, she was looking forward to having a Democrat back in the White House. Eight long years of Eisenhower's stagnant approach to medical research was quite enough. Over the next two days, she visited with acquaintances in high places to ask if they'd be supporting Stevenson. Mayor Robert Wagner of New York, Mayor Richard Daley of Chicago, NBC president Robert Kintner, and others all shook their heads. Their support was going to Kennedy. On July 13, the convention's third day, Kennedy gained a narrow majority of the voting delegates on the first ballot and was proclaimed the nominee. The following day, he announced Lyndon Johnson as his choice for running mate.

The Republican candidate and sitting vice president, Richard Nixon, had faced little opposition to succeed Eisenhower. But facing Kennedy fever was another matter. There were four debates scheduled between the candidates. These were not only the first televised debates ever conducted for a presidential election but also the turning point. Never before had Americans been able to compare their choices side by side, and from their living rooms. While Kennedy was tanned, vigorous, and confident, Nixon was pale, irritable, and sweating profusely. He looked significantly older than Kennedy, although in reality it was only by four years.

The election was exciting and incredibly close. "I really suffered," Mary later said, "because I thought Nixon would be a disaster of such unparalleled proportion that I didn't know what to do."

In the end, while Kennedy won the popular vote by less than one-fifth of a percentage point, he took the Electoral College, with the White House as his prize. During it all, Mary had learned two things. First, unlike her initial impression, she saw that Kennedy was very much presidential material. His looks had changed considerably during the campaign, and she thought he had become quite handsome. Second, she saw that Stevenson was not husband material, as some had suggested. His mood swings and indecisiveness during and after the campaign would never work for her in the long run.

The day before Kennedy's inauguration on Thursday, January 20, Washington was hit with a tremendous snowstorm. Eight inches fell on the city, cars were stranded, and Washington National Airport was shut down. But by noon on Friday, the city had been cleared and the sun shone. It was as bright a day as Truman's inauguration twelve years earlier, although with the wind chill, the temperature felt like seven degrees. Mary braved the cold in a white mink coat and matching hat, and then celebrated at the inaugural ball in a stunning blue brocade gown adorned with diamonds and pearls.

She was invited to Kennedy's White House for the first time on May 8, 1961. After a ceremony in which Kennedy congratulated astronaut Alan Shepard for his fifteen-minute trip into space (the first American to make that journey), she and Jackie visited Winterthur, the Delaware estate of Henry du Pont. Du Pont's keen eye and growing collection of early American furniture played perfectly into a project Jackie was planning: complete restoration of the White House. Mary's well-known love of art, culture, and beauty made her a perfect partner in this project. She was so inspired to get the ball rolling, she gave Jackie a $10,000 check on the plane ride back to Washington. It was the first of many donations.

The president invited Mary to return to the White House a month later. He wanted her to join the board of the National Cultural Center he was planning. In a country as large and as wealthy as the United States, Kennedy believed, such a center was long overdue. Mary was flattered by his offer, heartily agreeing with the concept of a cultural center. But the first board meetings were agony: they were disorganized and led by people who had no experience in fundraising. Their plans were too immense, and they were seeking too much money from a nation that had never thought of culture as a necessity.

Mary asked for another appointment with Kennedy. "I remember I came into the room on a lovely sort of warm day," she described. "He looked so handsome. He said, 'Well now, what is the problem?'" Mary couldn't bear to tell him what she really thought of the cultural board. And she couldn't very well turn down the first thing the new president asked of her, so she accepted. But she also figured that if she participated in his pet project, perhaps he'd be inclined to support hers. Jack Kennedy could very well be her new champion in medical research.

⁓

Dr. Kenneth Endicott, who had become the director of NCI in 1960, observed, "Basic virologists still look down their noses at cancer virologists. . . . [The disdain] is rooted in the view that the scientific problems are so insuperable, so little understood, that anyone involved in cancer research didn't have his head screwed on right."[3]

The source of the distance between cancer researchers and those in other disciplines is not difficult to trace. Prior to the last quarter of the twentieth century, cancer was the outlier in medical school education. Since little was understood about its cause or cure, medical students were taught only about its treatment and (if the patient survived) rehabilitation. Oncology wasn't a designated subspecialty of internal medicine in the United States until 1972. It was, therefore, only as the result of courageous, resilient, determined, and tireless individuals that the search for light in the darkness of cancer continued. Whether his head was "screwed on right" or not, Sidney Farber continued to be one of those. In fact, he was a shining star.

As Mary's relationship with him progressed from polite professionalism to real friendship, so did Farber's progress in chemotherapy. They exchanged countless letters, Farber's sometimes rambling. Together, they believed that a cure for cancer might not be far off. The doctor was so convinced that in a 1954 letter to Mary, he called their work a crusade. There it was: the word that had buzzed in Mary's heart and head since Albert's death.[4]

Farber's letters described not only his progress in chemotherapy but also progress in the various committees and organizations he and Mary had sprouted. NCI had seen the benefit of their idea to pool chemotherapy research. Together, they had organized the congressional lobby that created the Cancer Chemotherapy National Service Center (CCNSC) in April 1955. CCNSC would begin with a $5 million bank account, of which $4.2 million was earmarked for research grants. It was the first federal program promoting cancer drug discovery, and Dr. Endicott would take up the chief duties.

The chemicals being tested by CCNSC came from a plethora of sources. One, nitrogen mustard (commonly known as mustard gas), had been used as a chemical weapon against Allied forces during World War I. Fearing the same might occur during World War II, chemists began studying an antidote. The lethal attack they saw mustard gas launch on the blood system led other researchers to ponder whether it might have the same result on blood cancers. Digging around in nature's pantry, as Farber had with his study of folic acid, they found that the rosy periwinkle flower contained alkaloids that killed cancer cells. The drug vincristine, another star in early chemotherapy, was the result. Every success supported the words of American writer and biochemistry professor Isaac

Asimov: "The most exciting phrase to hear in science, the one that heralds new discoveries, is not 'Eureka!' but 'That's funny . . . '"

There was real debate, however, as to whether these new cancer drugs were doing more harm than good. Some physicians viewed the administration of "poisons" to those already near death as barbaric, even though they—or their parents—had agreed to the clinical trials. The newly dubbed "chemotherapists" (those who administered the drugs) became known as the "lunatic fringe." Chemotherapy research was revolutionary, and therefore controversial. Thick skin was a requirement for these researchers, as it was for Mary.[5]

Thick skin appeared to be paying off, however. In fiscal 1962, Congress appropriated the unheard-of sum of $43.7 million for chemotherapy research (over $400 million in today's money). Yet that same year, 361,810 Americans—more than the entire population of Fort Worth, Texas—would die of cancer. The "lunatic fringe" would have to work harder and faster.

—

The most beautiful house on the French Riviera was owned by (according to some) the most beautiful woman in the world. Enid, Lady Kenmare, outlived four husbands, was enriched by each, and is a story unto herself. Enid's third husband bought her a magnificent thirty-room mansion in the town of Saint-Jean-Cap-Ferrat. Called La Fiorentina, it was the color of ripe peaches, and situated on its own seven-acre peninsula jutting out into the Mediterranean. Having homes all over the world, Enid leased out the mansion for six weeks every summer. For over a decade Mary was her tenant, those weeks in France being the only spans of time she allowed herself a respite from the crusade.[6]

Two swimming pools, glorious architecture, and a dozen bedrooms made La Fiorentina an entertainment epicenter. Guests arrived like an exotic caravan. Friends from New York made sure to pay a visit during their own European holidays. Congressmen and doctors stopped by en route to international meetings. Actors made their way from Hollywood. Prince Rainier and Princess Grace came from neighboring Monaco for parties. And nearly every summer, Gerald

Van der Kamp was a guest. As the curator of Versailles, he was also the fellow who had suggested Albert and Danny Kaye climb up to the palace roof. Mary's high-profile friends were the talk of Cap-Ferrat every summer, gossip that one year made it to the ears of a cat burglar.

On August 28, 1961, in a scene straight out of *To Catch a Thief*, the burglar slipped from La Fiorentina's roof into a second-story bedroom. While Mary and her guests were occupied on the terrace with champagne and breathtaking Mediterranean views, the thief made off with $180,000 in jewels ($1.7 million today), along with Van der Kamp's passkeys to every door in Versailles. Other thefts occurred in the neighborhood that summer as well, bringing the grand total to over $1 million in furs, jewelry, and cash ($9.6 million today). No one was ever caught.[7]

Despite that episode, Mary adored her European escapes. They served a very useful purpose as well: to select her wardrobe for the next year. She wasn't fond of shopping, so she did it with dispatch. Since Lake Como, Italy, was just three hundred miles from Cap-Ferrat, and the little towns surrounding the lake were famous for their luscious silk, Mary stayed at the Villa del Balbianello during her wardrobe-hunting expeditions. The fourteenth-century lakefront monastery had been turned into an estate so fabulous, it was used as a setting for movies. But the roads surrounding the lake were treacherous. So Mary went by boat, a classic mahogany speedboat driven by her teenage nephew, Jim Fordyce. He gallantly guided his aunt from one town to another to make her purchases.

But it was the visits to the *maisons de la haute couture* of Paris that were the most fun. Sometimes at fashion shows, other times in salons, Mary selected items that suited both her figure—she was never satisfied with her weight—and her passion for the color blue. Friends thought she favored the color because it complemented her remarkable eyes; she said wearing hues of the same color made accessorizing easier. Colors, however, are also thought to signify personality traits. Light blue is associated with health and healing, while dark blue represents knowledge and integrity. Those words certainly paint an accurate picture of Mary. While she occasionally chose a shade of pink for evening gowns, blue and her omnipresent three strands of pearls were the daily uniform. Along with her always perfectly coiffed bouffant hair, no one would have guessed at the savvy and steely warrior beneath the veneer.

—

At Mary's urging, President Kennedy agreed to hold a conference on the diseases that were responsible for two out of every three deaths in America. Twenty-five doctors—all top in their fields—had come from across the country on April 17, 1961, to make recommendations to Kennedy on how to turn the tide against these diseases and save American lives. But the meeting was not to be. As the doctors were about to convene, Kennedy was occupied by what would become one of the worst military failures in American history. The president had agreed to send fifteen hundred American-trained Cuban fighters to overthrow the new Communist regime of Fidel Castro. When they landed in Cuba, on the shore of the Bay of Pigs, they were overwhelmed by local militia.[8] Kennedy spent the day locked up with his advisors, and the conference on the killer diseases was relegated to a back burner.

In truth, and unlike his Democratic predecessors, Kennedy wasn't much interested in increasing medical research funding. Although he had raised the NIH budget by $50 million in his first year, the amounts certainly weren't what Mary, Hill, and Fogarty were expecting, given the success they had had with President Truman. And while geopolitical events sometimes got in the way of the crusade, personal events often brought it to the fore. On December 19, 1961, Kennedy's seventy-three-year-old father suffered a stroke. He survived, but he was paralyzed on his right side and his speech was impaired. With the common ground of parents having suffered strokes, Mary tried a different approach when she met with Kennedy the following July. "I know what frustration you must have had finding that your father couldn't be substantially helped," she began sympathetically. Telling Kennedy many Americans felt the same way, she continued, "Practically nothing is being done about it. I think it would be wonderful if you would appoint a presidential commission on strokes."

The president readily agreed, and Mary was optimistic. What she didn't realize was that by this time, Kennedy had begun to see her in an entirely different light. She wasn't just a wealthy socialite with an interest in art. His brother Ted made that clear: "When I first came to the Senate [in 1962], I remember very clearly the advice that President Kennedy gave me. 'Have lunch with medical school professors, have dinner with Nobel Prize winners. But if you really want to know what needs to be done in medical research in America, have a talk with Mary Lasker.'"[9]

Being recognized in magazines as a woman of both poetry and power was all well and good, but Mary was always forced to add a significant dose of patience. Kennedy suggested that Mary take up the stroke commission idea with his advisors Ted Sorensen (White House counsel) and Mike Feldman (deputy special counsel). Gathering them together, however, was akin to herding cats. With such a full slate of campaign promises, the White House was in a near constant state of hyperactivity, and another meeting about the commission didn't gel until December. At that point Mary and Farber met with Sorensen and Feldman, who by this time had decided it would be best to avoid the appearance of creating a commission so closely related to events in the president's family.

Mary responded by rattling off the death toll from strokes the previous year, pointing out that strokes, along with cancer and heart disease, now accounted for three-quarters of American deaths. Thinking out loud, Feldman asked why they couldn't create a commission involving all three. It was a brilliant idea; Mary was thrilled. But seven more months passed before there was any action on that suggestion. "Hurry up and wait" was common when it came to moving the behemoth federal government.

On a return trip to the White House in July 1963, Mary finally got the chance to suggest the combined commission to Kennedy. "Well, I certainly agree with you," he told her. "Let's do it!" The president called in Feldman and told him to work with Mary on a list of potential commission members. At her urging, Dr. Michael DeBakey of Baylor University was selected to be chairman. Mary headed off for her European holiday, and when she returned in October, it was to the news that the commission would be announced in the last week of November.

"Mike is a man who puts Tabasco sauce on everything he eats—and everything he says." This colorful description from a friend of DeBakey's was pinpoint accurate. The man known as the "Texas Tornado" was the son of a Lebanese immigrant druggist and his wife. Born in Lake Charles, Louisiana, in 1908, DeBakey was inspired to become a physician from the doctors who visited his father's pharmacy. While in medical school at Tulane University in New Orleans, he took a part-time job in surgical research. Heart surgery at the time was nearly unknown; stopping the organ to repair it wasn't feasible. That fact motivated DeBakey to develop the roller pump that would one day become an integral part of the heart-lung machine, which would allow doctors to pause a beating heart for repair. And that was just the first of DeBakey's long list of incredible innovations.[10]

He earned a surgical fellowship, but World War II diverted his path. Joining the army, he went to work in the surgeon general's office. After the war, DeBakey moved his family to Houston, home of Baylor University's College of Medicine. He became chair of the Department of Surgery, where his passion and twenty-hour workdays produced lifesaving surgeries and devices, bringing him to worldwide attention. In April 1955, Albert Einstein's Princeton physician called DeBakey. The scientist had a ruptured abdominal blood vessel, and the doctor wondered if DeBakey's newly developed Dacron patch would work. DeBakey assured the doctor it would and that he should operate immediately. But Einstein refused the surgery, saying, "I want to go when I want. It is tasteless to prolong life artificially. I have done my share; it is time to go. I will do it elegantly." And he did, the following day.

By this time, of course, Mary knew all about Michael DeBakey, too. She had heard the stories of his boundless energy and remarkable skills. She had also heard about his irascibility during surgeries. He was never anything but a gentleman and friend to Mary, however. DeBakey was immensely impressed by her drive to increase funding for the very disease he was fighting. They had met when he joined the National Advisory Heart Council a few years after it was formed. DeBakey would later say of her, "Mary Lasker has done more than any other single individual in the country to improve our health." In mutual admiration, she found his insatiable curiosity for research not only thrilling but the perfect quality for a citizen witness to testify before Congress. He obliged, many times over.

Mary had made certain that DeBakey was among the twenty-five physicians ready to meet with Kennedy before their conference had been canceled two years earlier. Now, with someone this well known to chair the president's heart disease, cancer, and stroke commission, conquering those major killers looked certain. The commission would have its first meeting after the president came back from a tour of Texas.

～

At 12:30 p.m. Central Time on Friday, November 22, 1963, America was changed forever. While riding in a motorcade in Dallas and waving to a jubilant crowd, President Kennedy was shot. His limo sped the three and a half miles to the closest hospital, Parkland, but thirty minutes later the president was proclaimed dead. As shock waves spread out across the country and the world, a search for the assassin began. Less than two hours later, Lee Harvey Oswald was arrested for killing the president as well as a police officer as he was fleeing. The slain president's body was placed on Air Force One, while a grim-faced Vice President Johnson took the oath of office.

Oswald was charged with the murders of the Dallas police officer and President Kennedy. Two days later, at nearly the same moment the president had been shot, Oswald was being taken through the basement of the Dallas police headquarters on his way to the county jail. Television production didn't yet have delay mechanisms. As America watched, Oswald was shot in front of their eyes by Jack Ruby. Oswald, too, was taken to Parkland Hospital, where he died at almost the same time of day as President Kennedy had forty-eight hours earlier.

Despite the sting of losing the 1960 presidential election, Richard Nixon wrote to Mrs. Kennedy the day after the president's death: "While the hand of fate made Jack and me political opponents, I always cherished the fact that we were personal friends from the time we came to the Congress together in 1947."[11]

Mary reflected later on the progress they would have made against heart disease and cancer had Kennedy returned from Dallas. "We thought we'd have more time," she said. A grieving nation felt the same.

⁓

Lyndon Baines Johnson became a congressman from the tenth district of Texas in 1937. But he had set much loftier goals for himself, as his biographer Robert Caro observed: "Johnson's ambition was uncommon—in the degree to which it was unencumbered by even the slightest excess weight of ideology, of philosophy, of principles, of beliefs." After a first unsuccessful run for the Senate in 1941 and then a stint in the U.S. Navy during World War II, Johnson would try for the Senate again in the fall of 1948. First, however, he had to face down a rival Democrat in an August primary. Johnson won that race (some say dishonestly) by eighty-seven votes and went on to defeat the Republican challenger in November, earning the nickname "Landslide Lyndon."[12]

Mary didn't know anything about Johnson at the time of that election, but a Texas relative of Albert's was very enthused about him. "I was, in principle, for any Democrat against any Republican," Mary explained, "because by this time I was interested in health legislation. And I knew that the Democrats were much more generous-minded legislatively and financially than the Republicans." When Johnson became Senate majority leader in 1955, her friend Anna Rosenberg told her, "You'll never get anywhere in the Congress unless you get Lyndon Johnson on your side."[13] And Anna knew he would not be easy to convince. He wanted facts on issues, and after Mary presented them, he verified them with doctors and scientists.

LBJ had been disappointed that Mary didn't support his presidential aspirations in 1960, but he respected her loyalty to Stevenson. Once the Kennedy-Johnson ticket had formed, Mary was more than generous with a $50,000 donation (nearly half a million dollars today). Not only had Mary gotten Johnson on her side, as Anna had suggested, but he became her strongest advocate for health research and education. In the spring of 1961, while Mary was having lunch at Romanoff's on Rodeo Drive in Beverly Hills, she was told that the Johnson Moving Company wanted to speak with her on the telephone.

"You must be mistaken," she told the mâitre d'; "I don't know them." The mâitre d' went to verify the caller and returned to tell Mary it was Mr. Johnson. "Is it *Vice President* Johnson?" The frazzled mâitre d' didn't know, so Mary went to the phone. It was indeed the vice president, who was calling to ask her to serve on his Commission for Equal Employment Opportunities, an effort to eliminate prejudice in hiring practices. She protested that she didn't know anything about hiring, but he insisted. "I thought, 'Well, I need Lyndon, so I'd better say yes,'" she recounted. "And I said yes."

Mary and the Johnsons saw each other off and on during the Kennedy administration, and she and Lady Bird Johnson became very close. As had been the case when Roosevelt died, Mary would once again live through a historic presidential transition. Both JFK and LBJ were on her mind the morning after the assassination when she called Senator Hubert Humphrey, whose campaigns she had also supported. She wanted to share an epiphany she had had during the night. Given the former president's interest in the creation of the National Cultural Center, she felt it should be renamed the Kennedy Center for the Performing Arts. Would Humphrey take the suggestion to Congress and ask them to give money to begin building it immediately? Humphrey thought it was a terrific idea and promised he would get the ball rolling.

Mary next asked about Johnson. "How is he? Have you seen him?" Humphrey said that, in fact, Johnson had called him and said, "Hubert, go to your office and call up all of our friends. Let them know that we need their help." Not surprisingly, Mary was on that list, and Johnson himself called her later that evening to express the same sentiment. "It must have been a series of several hundred calls that he made saying, 'I want your support. I need your help,'" she described. "There's nothing more touching than the President of the United States saying this to an innocent citizen who is sitting at home."

"When are you coming down here?" the president asked Mary.

"I'm coming tomorrow for the funeral," Mary told him.

"Come to dinner when you get here," Johnson requested.

A small, somber group gathered the night of November 25, including the son of Texas governor John Connally, who had also been riding in Kennedy's car; the governor had been seriously wounded but was recovering. Mary sat next to the new president and told him about renaming the cultural center. He liked the idea and said he'd get a staff member on it immediately. News of that kind traveled fast in Washington, and by the next day bills for the new Kennedy Center were presented to both the House and the Senate.

Johnson had assured Mary he would see her "at any time, any place," and Mary took him up on it a few weeks later, on December 4, when she returned to Washington. After chatting about the Kennedy Center, she brought up the heart disease, cancer, and stroke commission that had been in the works during the Kennedy years. Johnson was intrigued, which wasn't surprising considering his near-fatal heart attack eight years earlier. He called in Abe Fortas, his friend, attorney, and later an associate Supreme Court justice. Fortas told Johnson it was a terrific idea and that Mary was absolutely on the right track, particularly, as Mary had pointed out, because Johnson would become the first president to undertake a formal attack on these killers. Insomuch as Johnson had left nearly all of Kennedy's staff in place, Mike Feldman was next to receive news that the commission was moving forward. This was good news to him, too, as he had already climbed on the bandwagon for it. The commission inched toward the finish line.

The next day, Herbert Lehman died. Lehman, a former governor of New York and later a senator from the state, had been a friend to both Mary and the Johnsons. After LBJ's heart attack, Lehman had asked the Senate to stand in silent prayer for him. The new president would never forget the meaningful gesture. Lady Bird called Mary to ask her if, since they would be coming to New York for Lehman's funeral, she would come back to Washington with them. Mary agreed and cleared her calendar.

After the funeral, Mary and the Johnsons traveled to Idlewild Airport (which would be renamed John F. Kennedy International Airport later that month) and then on to the capital. They landed at Andrews Air Force Base, and a helicopter took them to the White House lawn. As she walked into the foyer that rainy, chilly evening, Mary realized it was just the second night the Johnsons would sleep in the executive mansion, having moved in the day before. Mary remembered, "We walked into this house, at this time, all draped in black. We walked around, talking in whispers. It was one the saddest things I've ever done in my life." Mary would be the Johnsons' very first overnight guest.[14] She spent the night in the Queen's Bedroom, which had been redone during Jackie's beautiful White House renovation.

Like all other vice presidential families up until this point, the Johnsons didn't have a designated home. Right after the 1960 election, they had purchased a three-story mansion named The Elms, located on 52nd Street NW. They had remained in that house after LBJ was sworn in, wanting to give Jackie Kennedy ample time to relocate. Part of the motivation for Lady Bird's invitation to Mary was to take her to The Elms the next day to decide what among the china, decor, paintings, and other possessions should be packed and stored and what should be brought to the White House.

When they arrived the next morning, Mary saw that much of the furniture had already been moved into Lady Bird's White House rooms and those of her daughters (Lynda, nineteen, and Luci, sixteen). She and Lady Bird had the breakable things, including a set of plates and mugs that Mary had given her, wrapped and boxed. Everything was then loaded into the waiting car, along with a selection of paintings, and they returned to the White House to arrange them. Lady Bird had visited Mary's home in New York; she knew what a deft eye her friend had when it came to artwork. Deciding which paintings should be hung where and how was right up Mary's alley, and she gladly obliged.

The next day, the two trooped to the West Wing to make decisions on what the president's office needed. Mary was shocked at how empty the Oval Office looked. The room was entirely different from when she had last seen it, while visiting Kennedy the summer before. It had been in the midst of a makeover, to be done while Kennedy was on that fateful Texas trip. The paintings and statues that had been there on loan from the National Gallery had been returned. Now there were only two sofas, the desk, and Johnson's rocking chair, similar to Kennedy's. It was truly a tabula rasa.

The general consensus was that a selection of Southwest-themed art would be most to the president's liking. But before any further discussion could take place, a wave of people descended on the office. The decorating would have to be tabled. There were 189.2 million Americans waiting to see how the new president would heal the nation.

Chapter 9

"It's Just Piddling"

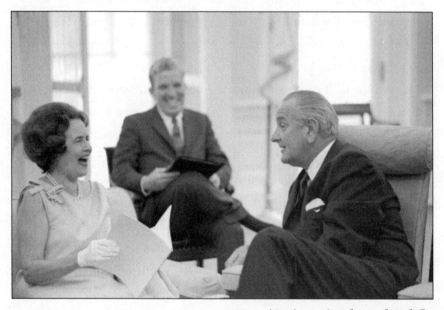

Mary and President Lyndon Johnson in the Oval Office, as Johnson's special assistant Douglass Cater looks on, circa 1960s.

"Good evening, I'm Ed Murrow. And the name of the program is *Person to Person*. It's all live—there's no film."[1]

The knowledge and conviction that Mary would bring to President Johnson's Commission on Heart Disease, Cancer, and Stroke in the early 1960s had been honed by events like this 1959 television appearance. It was the first time she had appeared on television, and she was quite excited to be a guest of this broadcasting pioneer.

It is important to remember that television of this era no more resembles today's version of the medium than a 1959 Cadillac resembles a 2023 Tesla. We now access up-to-the-second information on every topic at any hour. But if those who actually owned a television in 1959 hoped it might provide a diversion for insomnia, they were out of luck. Networks (there were just three) signed on at six in the morning and, after playing "The Star-Spangled Banner," signed off at midnight. All this goes to say that the dearth of programming made Murrow's innovative show more remarkable and, by extension, more entertaining.

The show's setup was remarkably similar to a modern-day Zoom meeting. Television viewers watched Murrow—never without a Camel cigarette—seated comfortably in his New York studio. Celebrities appeared on an enormous screen facing him as he interviewed them in their homes. On this particular Friday evening in 1959, after his customary opening, Murrow continued, "Mrs. Albert D. Lasker is a woman of many and varied interests: flowers and philanthropy, cancer research and community welfare." And on Murrow's enormous screen, Mary stood at the foot of the staircase in her Beekman Place home, wearing a smile, a large diamond brooch pinned to her dark dress, and her pearls. In answering one of Murrow's questions about current cancer treatment, Mary unleashed one of her most powerful weapons: expressing facts in terms anyone could understand. "The amount of money that's being spent for medical research, well it's just piddling," she declared. "You won't believe this: less is spent on cancer research than we spend on chewing gum!"[2]

When Mary rewatched the show four years later, she was once again reminded of how much her crusade was built on Albert's brilliant tutoring. Because of him, she was adept at molding public opinion, had honed the art of persuasion, employed strategic thinking, and had learned how to play the long game. Those skills were turning out results. When Mary and Florence first began their lobbying efforts in the mid-1940s, NIH's federal appropriation was less than $3 million. By the time of her appearance on Murrow's show, its funding was a whopping $560 million. It would inch toward, and finally hit, the $1 billion mark before the 1960s were over.

It had taken more than the citizen lobbyists' skills to enlarge the NIH coffers; they had allies there as well. In the early 1950s it was NIH director Dr. William Sebrell. His reaction to the increases in funding was simple: "I am not going to violate the wishes of Congress. If Congress says that they want the bulk of the money spent on cancer or neurology, or what have you, then that is where the money is going."[3] Unfortunately, Sebrell resigned after five years, feeling responsible for a horrible accident at Cutter Pharmaceuticals: the company was producing the new polio vaccine by inactivating live polio virus, but vials were misplaced and more than a hundred thousand children were injected with the live virus.[4] It fell to Surgeon General Scheele to select a new director. He found Dr. James Shannon to be the perfect candidate. A physician and physiologist, Shannon had been an NIH associate director in charge of research at the newly created National Heart Institute. It all looked so promising.

But as time passed, Mary developed a different opinion. She believed Shannon had been so seriously scarred by the fallout from the Cutter incident that he was ultra-cautious and moved agonizingly slowly in every endeavor. On top of that, just like Florence, Shannon was in the basic-research camp (focusing on advancing general knowledge), as opposed to Mary's preferred applied research. She later surmised, "He realized that if you talked about basic research, very few people could judge whether you were making any progress or not. Whereas, if you were interested in clinical research . . . it would be clear whether you were failing or succeeding."

Yet for Shannon to continue receiving NIH funding and for Mary to achieve her research goals, each realized they needed the other. Plus, Dr. Scheele—of whom Mary thought highly, and who returned the sentiment—had given Shannon his stamp of approval. Thus, they forged ahead in an interesting alliance during what came to be known as the "golden era" of NIH.[5]

The first part of the alliance was the research lobby, which was widely given credit for waking the country up to the need for medical research. Mary may have been its titular head, but the group was much more than just her, as she was always quick to point out. Florence, Gorman, Farber, DeBakey, and myriad others played critical roles. While Mary would speak with Shannon only a few times and visit his office just once during the thirteen years he headed NIH, the others acted as Mary's proxies, conveying the crusade's message.

The second part of the alliance consisted of Fogarty and Hill, chairs of their respective appropriations subcommittees. They welcomed and respected the enthusiasm, expertise, and power of the group that had come to be known as the "Laskerites." And they paved the way forward in growing the NIH budget. When conflicts over issues arose with the Laskerites and Shannon sought help from the legislators, Hill usually suggested a letter or memo expressing alternatives as a compromise. Fogarty, on the other hand, preferred a good drink with fellow Irishman Shannon; whiskey made hammering things out much easier. Regardless of which man Shannon sought help from, they served brilliantly as the crusade's—and Mary's—emissaries.[6]

Filling the role of the alliance's third part was Shannon himself. He recognized that if NIH hadn't had the support of both the citizen lobby and Congress and hadn't been given the chance to grow, it would have been relegated to a minor division of PHS after World War II. There was never a question that Shannon wanted to find a cure for cancer and the other conditions that plagued his fellow humans. But his cautious nature won out. That was evident when he chose this quote from the French writer Voltaire for his speech at the annual meeting of the Association of American Medical Colleges: "Doctors pour drugs, of which they know little, for diseases, of which they know less, into human beings, about whom they know nothing."[7]

Shannon's position was the same one that many biomedical scientists held. Problems had to be attacked carefully, systematically. Gaps in knowledge of genetics, biochemistry, molecular biology, biophysics, immunology, and so on must be filled before proceeding. This position prompted Farber, who was testifying in the House one day, to say that "medical scientists still do not totally understand the mechanism of aspirin, insulin, and antihypertension [blood pressure] drugs," and yet those drugs were saving humans from suffering and death.[8] That "gaps in knowledge" argument would hound Mary for years.

In the short term, however, she and her lobbyists developed a sound work-around. When Congress allocated funds to NIH, it now added language clearly directing the institutes on the use of those funds and the pace of the research. A Senate committee report clearly illustrates this tactic: "The committee . . . directs that expansion of clinical investigation [in chemotherapy] proceed as rapidly as the clinical and scientific resources of the country permit." That still didn't stop Mary from grumbling, "Too many of them are without a deep sense of urgency."

⟶

When Mary had prayed for a baby sister nearly six decades earlier—and then proclaimed at her birth that her name would be Alice—she could never have imagined the important role her little sister would fill. Alice had moved to New York City as soon as she graduated from Smith College in 1928, and never left. After a stint in fashion publicity at Lord and Taylor, she worked in public relations at the new Rockefeller Center. Once she married Al Fordyce in 1939, she left that position. But like Mary, Alice never stopped working.

True sisters in crime, Alice and Mary had all the good elements of a sibling relationship, and very few of the bad ones. Mary felt special affection for Alice's only child, Jim. Now that Mary was widowed, with no children of her own, the three Fordyces became an integral part of Mary's life. Alice was more than willing to roll up her sleeves and dive into whatever Mary needed. She was a part of the beautification projects, served as secretary of Mary's Committee on National Health, and would hold the same role when it evolved into the National Health Education Committee. She was also the vice chairman of the National Committee on Mental Health and, when needed, served as a citizen witness.

It was work on the Albert and Mary Lasker Foundation, however, that gave Alice the greatest pleasure. Mary had expanded the foundation's name to include their first names soon after Albert's death. At the same time, she renamed the awards the Albert Lasker Medical Research Awards, wanting in both cases to make certain her beloved husband, the man who made it all possible, was never forgotten. Mary then became the foundation president, and Alice was happy to step up as executive vice president. Just as her brother-in-law had done, Alice preferred being in the background of the foundation. That didn't mean, however, that she wouldn't speak up when called to do so. As the awareness of the awards grew, the ceremonies became large productions. Recipients had to be instructed as to what was expected of them. One said of Alice, "Both myself and many other scientists, more stubborn, busier, and with all their own prior engagements, have found it impossible to escape being organized by this lady. She is an absolutely irresistible force."[9] Being an "irresistible force" was a family trait.

Nearly as important as the awards themselves were the presentation venues. Their selection, the menus, and the table settings had to exude the air of respect and sophistication due them, something for which the Woodard sisters became famous. The awards hopscotched from one hotel to another across Manhattan. And just as with Mary's personal social events, the attendees and presenters were a who's who of politics, Hollywood, and medicine.

Albert's original dream of giving seed money that could grow big had done just that: the winners' names became familiar to Americans. And the discoveries for which they were recognized went on to save millions of lives around the world, which, in turn, inspired other researchers. By 1964, fifteen of the Lasker Award winners had gone on to win Nobel Prizes. No wonder they became known as the "American Nobels." The categories continued to increase along with the award amounts. Added to basic and clinical research awards were recognition in medical journalism, public service, and special achievement.

The single element that didn't vary from year to year was the inscribed statuette that Alice presented to the recipients: golden replicas of the famed Winged Victory of Samothrace. The actual statue, discovered in Greece in the nineteenth century, is a headless, armless figure of a woman, created to honor a Greek sea victory. She was meant to convey a sense of action and triumph, both certainly unequivocal goals of medical research.

Like Mary, Alice often gave credit to their mother for the direction of her life's path. "It's true that she was extraordinarily persuasive—a seller of dreams, really," Alice reminisced. "But she also had very good ideas. And they were not selfish ideas. They were ideas to help others."[10] Sara Woodard's daughters certainly lived up to the model she had carved.

~

Two and a half weeks before the 1964 Albert Lasker Awards were presented, President Lyndon Johnson had reclaimed his nickname as "Landslide Lyndon" with a reelection victory. But the road to get there had not been easy. LBJ and Lady Bird entered the White House as a result of the televised murder of an extremely popular president, who became a charismatic martyr. And while Johnson had insisted on carrying out all of JFK's plans, like Truman he never felt he was a legitimate president, someone the nation *wanted* in that office. He and the First Lady had spent many hours discussing what their next steps should be. Often plagued by self-doubt, Johnson relied heavily on his wife for advice. Facing him (or the next president, should it not be him) was a Communist threat in Southeast Asia, racial distress, and a poverty level that was a disgrace for the nation. Johnson needed a plan, *his* plan.

Words play a crucial role in politics. Bad words are deadly to a career, but good words, even if they're accidental, can make the sun shine. And often, presidents' speechwriters keep an ongoing list of words and phrases to plug in as needed. Robert Goodwin had joined Kennedy's speechwriting team in 1959 and stayed on when Johnson became president. In crafting the 1964 State of the Union address, the president and Goodwin included the idea of "declaring war" on poverty, an issue over which LBJ was highly distraught. The press liked Johnson's reference to a "war on poverty," so the president reiterated the phrase as he toured the nation. Then, delivering a speech in Chicago at a Democratic fundraising dinner on April 24, Johnson spoke of keeping a Democrat in the White House when election day rolled around in November. He told the audience that if the party helped build "a great society of the highest order, we do not have to worry about success at the polls."[11]

Goodwin trotted out the term "great society" a number of times in the ensuing weeks, including in a speech Johnson gave at Ohio State University the Thursday before Mother's Day. The president told students, "To you of this student body, I say merely as a statement of fact: America is yours—yours to make a better land, yours to build the great society."[12] But it wasn't until graduation day at the University of Michigan, on May 22, that the press caught on. Speaking to the ninety thousand assembled in the football stadium that warm morning, Johnson said, "I intend to establish working groups to prepare a series of conferences and meetings. . . . From these studies, we will begin to set our course toward a great society."[13]

Like an explosion in ink, newspaper headlines across the country screamed the phrase. Franklin Roosevelt—whom Johnson idolized—had had his New Deal. Kennedy's New Frontier had been stopped short by his assassination. Now, Johnson had an agenda to which he would forever be connected, the Great Society. The timing was no mistake. LBJ and Lady Bird had decided just nine days earlier that he would, indeed, seek reelection in November.

Mary was beyond happy; she genuinely liked the Johnsons, both as individuals and as leaders. Her relationship with LBJ had been solidified in 1959, when he was still Senate majority leader. Mary had gone to see him about supporting Lister Hill in his presentation of the "citizens' budget" for medical research on the Senate floor. Johnson wanted to know what he was asking for. When Mary told him $78 million for fiscal 1960, he was shocked and asked her, "Isn't that too much?" She shot back, "Not if you want to live." Johnson took a breath, then asked her to write a speech for him to deliver after Hill presented the bill. A savvy politician, LBJ knew the impact of Mary's support of the candidates he needed as allies. Furthermore, Mary's affection for Lady Bird warmed the president's heart. And Lady Bird returned the affection. In her diary, the First Lady praised Mary for her ability to bring out in LBJ "the oddest combination of cynicism and undying belief in the mind of man." And then she added, "Mary herself is so smart."[14]

Mary believed in Johnson's war on poverty. "Poverty makes disease," she said, "and disease makes poverty." His work in civil rights (which culminated in the Civil Rights Act being signed into law on July 2, 1964) would go far in healing national wounds. But his overarching Great Society would be the perfect incubator for the kind of successes in medical research Mary had long dreamed of. First, however, there was an election to win.

Steely-jawed Phoenix conservative senator Barry Goldwater had won the Republican nomination at the party's convention in July. Now it was August, and the Democrats would have their turn in Atlantic City. Johnson's was the only name considered for president. Minnesota senator Hubert Humphrey was considered likely to fill the vice president's office, which had been vacant since the assassination. There would be no televised debates, but there was a great deal of tough campaigning ahead, with Johnson's Great Society continuing to take shape. On October 16, he delivered a speech at a Liberal Party rally, held in Madison Square Garden. Mary attended, of course, sitting in the wing of the stage. Johnson warned about changing administrations at this point in time, given the ever-looming Communist threat throughout the world. Taking a stab at Goldwater's hawkish stand on defense, Johnson told the crowd a Goldwater victory would "put in danger the safety of our country and the world's hopes for peace."[15]

Then the president switched gears and, spotting Mary in the wing, spoke in that direction. "And we are going to eliminate cancer, heart disease, and stroke, just as we have polio." There was an audible gasp in the arena. Had the president just promised to cure cancer? Since January, Mary had hammered home the need to eradicate those diseases. Now she and everyone else in the country knew he was committed to the fight.

Three hundred forty-four days after Lyndon Johnson had been put into office by an assassin's bullet, he won on his own accord, taking forty-four states plus the District of Columbia and 61 percent of the popular vote. Mary called the Johnsons at their Texas ranch the next day to congratulate them. Lady Bird told her, "If you have any ideas of things that I should do, tell me." Mary promised she would, and met with the First Lady a few weeks later to talk about possibilities for the inauguration. Above all, she told Lady Bird, it must be "memorable, and different from other inaugurations, to mark the beginning of his Great Society." And it was.

The actual inauguration was January 20, but the celebration began two days before. Mary arrived in Washington on the seventeenth and attended the inaugural gala the next night. Held in the Armory, as Kennedy's had been, it was quite the star-studded affair. Alfred Hitchcock served as master of ceremonies, and Barbra Streisand, Harry Belafonte, Julie Andrews, Carol Burnett, and others entertained. On the eighteenth was the inaugural concert, which Mary had agreed to co-chair with Abe Fortas and his wife. Held at Constitution Hall, it featured esteemed musicians Van Cliburn and Isaac Stern along with the National Symphony Orchestra.

Following the concert, everyone made their way to the State Department for what became known as "the greatest party of the Great Society." Mary (who wrote the check) and the Fortases hosted five hundred guests for dinner and dancing in honor of the president. The "elegant, candle-lit, floral-ornamented" rooms were done precisely to Mary's specifications. Masses of red and white carnations topped every surface and overflowed every vase. "If the great artists of our age can take time to give their talents, the least I can do is make the setting as enchanting and the party for them as gay as possible," Mary promised a reporter on the day of the party.[16]

"There was such a mixture of people," she remembered a few months later. "People who were part of the government, artists, writers, and people who were just social. Everyone was going around in a pleasant daze of champagne, seeing people they'd never seen before. Especially the president of the United States and his wife, very casually wandering around." Her escort that night—and to all of the inauguration festivities—was her nephew, Jim. He made the dinner even more memorable, and made newspaper stories the next day, by dancing the Watusi with the president's daughter Luci.

Inauguration day dawned bright and sunny but freezing. Mary had caught a cold, so she listened to the ceremony on the radio. But she rallied for the inaugural ball, dressed in a pink gown and long coat by Balenciaga. With four thousand in attendance, however, it was so crowded it was impossible to dance, eat, drink, or even carry on a conversation. Fortunately, she and the Fortases had planned a little party of their own, with another five hundred guests. Then, as it was for

Cinderella, the red carpets were rolled up and the ball gowns were packed away. It was time for Mary to get busy crafting her portion of the Great Society.

—

Exactly one year before his 1965 inauguration, Johnson had told the South Vietnamese government, "The United States will continue to furnish you and your people with the fullest measure of support in this bitter fight."[17] But in truth, the Vietnamese people were tired of foreigners. For nearly a century, the French had occupied the country, and amid the drama of World War II, a national independence coalition was born in Vietnam: the Viet Minh. Anti-Japanese and anti-French, the coalition was led by Ho Chi Minh.

In the postwar reorganization of Asia, the Viet Minh redoubled their efforts against the French. They were given both sheltered bases and heavy weapons by their newly formed neighbor to the north, the People's Republic of China. Using guerrilla tactics, the Viet Minh attacked until the French ultimately gave up in 1954. Then, as had just been done in Korea, the country was divided into north and south. That wasn't the Viet Minh's plan, and they began focusing their guerrilla attacks on South Vietnamese targets. The ongoing hostilities prompted Johnson, then Senate minority leader, to allude to the "domino effect," saying, "Today it is Indochina. Tomorrow, Asia may be in flames. And the day after, the Western Alliance may be in ruins."[18]

America ignored the history lesson it might have learned from the French. As the Cold War between the United States and the Soviet Union grew chillier, Eisenhower—who had coined the domino theory—sent seven hundred military personnel, along with economic aid, to the government of South Vietnam. Soon after becoming president, Kennedy quickly authorized sending an additional five hundred Special Forces and military advisors to assist the pro-Western South Vietnamese government. By the end of 1962, there were approximately eleven thousand U.S. military advisors in the region.

After Kennedy's assassination, the new president unhappily inherited the problem of this far-off and little-understood country. He told Henry Cabot Lodge Jr., ambassador to South Vietnam, "I am not going to lose Vietnam. I am not going to be the president who saw Southeast Asia go the way China went." Johnson had kept all of Kennedy's national security team intact, including the secretary of defense, Robert McNamara. "I feel like a jackass in a Texas hailstorm," he told McNamara. "I can't run, I can't hide and I can't make it stop." Then, on August 2, 1964, another option developed.[19]

The USS *Maddox* was attacked in the Gulf of Tonkin, off Vietnam's northern coast, by North Vietnamese torpedo boats. Two days later, American radar detected another attack. Whether or not the second was widely exaggerated, if not fabricated (as retrospective analysis suggests), Johnson ordered air strikes on North Vietnamese patrol boat bases. As the Viet Minh morphed into the Viet Cong, it appeared as though the "conflict" in Vietnam was becoming political quicksand, and a possible threat to Johnson's Great Society. War would continue to weave its tentacles through the crusade.

—

One night Mary received a phone call from the White House. "Listen," President Johnson said, "I got something I need for you to do for me."

"What is it?" she replied good-naturedly. "I'll do it if I can." Never in her wildest dreams could she have imagined what came next.

"I want to make you ambassador to Finland," Johnson told her.

Mary was in shock. "Oh my God, I can't move to Finland!"

Johnson insisted she'd be perfect for the job. "Right on the border of Russia," he said. "I need someone who's got some brains and some charm."

It was a ridiculous notion. Give up her home, her friends, and New York City and move halfway around the world? Going to France every summer was one thing. This was quite another. "Lyndon, I wouldn't be good!" Mary told him, frantically grasping for a reason he'd accept. The only thing that came to mind was the subject that was *always* on her mind. "I've got to get the answer to the different kinds of cancer," she insisted. He told her not to be hasty, to think it over for twenty-four hours.[20]

Mary really didn't need the time, but she agreed to speak with him again the next day, when she politely repeated that the ambassadorship was out of the question. But she reminded him of the memo she had sent earlier. It contained all the ingredients for his upcoming announcement of the creation of the Commission on Heart Disease, Cancer, and Stroke. He had promised to make the announcement in his health message to Congress on February 10, which he did.

"Cancer, heart disease, and strokes stubbornly remain the leading causes of death in the United States," the president said in that message. "I am establishing a Commission on Heart Disease, Cancer, and Strokes to recommend steps to reduce the incidence of these diseases through new knowledge and more complete utilization of the medical knowledge we already have."[21] His words were almost exactly what Mary had written for him.

She had also given Johnson her recommendations for commission members. Those included the many friends who had served in other capacities of the crusade. DeBakey would be chair, and commission members included Farber, former RCA president David Sarnoff, Emerson Foote, and Dr. Howard Rusk. Mary was back in Washington on Valentine's Day to discuss it all further. "I think you should have the names of more women for the commission," LBJ told her. "Get me more names of women!" So they added Bess Truman, Dr. Marion Fay (former president and dean of the Woman's Medical College of Pennsylvania), Dr. Jane Wright (associate professor of surgical research at New York University School of Medicine, and the commission's only African American), and Florence Mahoney.

Johnson wanted to know why Mary hadn't suggested herself for the commission. There was no need: she had handpicked the members, most of whose thoughts about medical research mirrored hers. She would be advised of the final report before it was presented, at which time she could add anything she felt might be lacking. Plus, she and her staff would be heavy contributors of statistics for the report.

The president good-naturedly accused her of simply wanting others to do the heavy lifting. "You can make more work for more people than anybody I've ever heard of," he teased. He still acknowledged her publicly, later saying that he appointed the commission "at the insistence of this lovely lady, Mary Lasker."[22] This would be the first time ever a president had ordered that direct aim be taken at solving the mysteries of America's three major killers. It was a step closer to Mary's dream of eradicating them forever.

Johnson was pleased with the suggestion of DeBakey as chair. The surgeon was a Texas Democrat *and* a heart specialist, two things that mattered to the president. DeBakey was genuinely honored and readily accepted, arriving at the White House on March 7 for the commission's official introduction to the public. Speaking with DeBakey ahead of time, Johnson told him he felt the most important task before the commission was to make recommendations that would improve doctors' ability to deal with heart disease, cancer, and strokes. How long would it take to complete the study? the president wanted to know. DeBakey, staggered by the enormousness of it all, suggested a year. That was not good enough for the president; Johnson wanted it completed before the 1965 State of the Union address. That was just nine months away, but the inspiring, off-the-cuff pep talk the president then gave the entire group of commission members made it seem possible. "Unless we do better," Johnson said, "two-thirds of all Americans now living will suffer or die from cancer, heart disease or stroke. I expect you to do something about it."[23]

The commission divided itself into subcommittees for each of the conditions, plus five other committees to support the overall work. From the outset, the cancer subcommittee was in agreement on the direction they wanted to go. Chaired by Farber, it also included Dr. Lee Clark, director and surgeon-in-chief of M. D. Anderson Hospital and Tumor Institute, and Dr. Frank Horsfall, president and director of the Sloan Kettering Institute for Cancer Research. Among other things, they strongly favored the creation of regional cancer centers that would become the hubs of scientific and clinical work, with "the eradication of cancer [as] the accepted institutional goal."

Working from the Executive Office Building, the commission was supplied with space and a support staff provided by PHS and NIH. They collected testimonies from national organizations (like ACS and the American Heart Association) and interviewed dozens of other expert witnesses in science and medicine. They analyzed the information and distilled it down to a hundred-plus-page document. "Report to the President: A National Program to Conquer

Heart Disease, Cancer and Stroke" was formally submitted to Johnson on December 9, 1964.

The original purpose of the commission was to bridge the gap between clinical research in the three diseases and the delivery of the results to actual patients. Of the thirty-five recommendations made in the report, the "national network for patient care [and] research teaching in heart disease, cancer and stroke" got the most attention. It recommended the creation of centers, spread across universities, hospitals, and research institutes. Within five years, there would be twenty-five heart centers, twenty cancer centers, and fifteen stroke centers, plus 150 diagnostic and treatment centers for heart conditions, 200 for cancer, and 100 for stroke. The whole thing became known as the Regional Medical Programs (RMP). The cost of implementing these recommendations would be $357 million in the first year and $739 million by the fifth year, for a total of $2.9 billion.

That amount, however, was put into perspective by the report's opening letter from DeBakey: "Our stated goals are neither impartial nor visionary—they *can* be achieved if we so will it. They *must* be achieved if we are to check the heavy losses these three diseases inflict upon our economy—close to $40 billion each year in lost productivity and lost taxes due to premature disability and death."[24]

This had always been one of Mary's greatest themes, of course. If medical research achieves its goals and lives are saved, society is better off in myriad ways, not the least of which comes in the form of cold, hard cash. But that point was missed by the newspaper headlines, which latched on to the overall cost: "$3 Billion War on Cancer, Heart Disease, Stroke Urged." The commission's report was quoted as saying that "emphasis should be placed locally for the provision of care for medically indigent patients in a diagnostic and treatment unit. Patients other than the medically indigent should pay for services."[25] Readers, however, saw that as federally funded medical care. In other words, the commission seemed to be advocating two of the dirtiest words in the English language: socialized medicine. The public was aghast; so was the American Medical Association.

In a brilliant political move, Mary and the president had originally included on the commission Dr. Hugh Hussey, the AMA's director of scientific activities.

In September, however, midway through the commission's work, Hussey had handed in his resignation, stating that the commission's direction was in potential conflict with AMA policy. That conflict was made clearer in a statement the association released the day after the debut of the recommendations. It had not had time to study the report, the association said. But it wanted to make clear that it would continue to oppose all federal intervention in the field of medicine.

Johnson was able to include the commission's report in his State of the Union address, as he'd hoped. It was the first evening speech to be carried live on all three television networks. Three days later, the president delivered a health message to Congress. How wonderful it would have been if the message had focused solely on the commission's recommendations. The president did, indeed, ask Congress to approve them. But the sweeping message also dealt with "hospital insurance for the elderly," commonly referred to as Medicare.

Sixteen days later, the legislative process to approve the commission's recommendations began. Bills were presented in both the House and the Senate, with Fogarty and Hill rolling up their sleeves to get the funds appropriated. But in the background, the AMA simmered. They would not be usurped again in their war to prevent socialized medicine, and used the next two months to continue to chip away at the DeBakey commission's recommendations.

When the October 6, 1965, signing of the Heart Disease, Cancer, and Stroke Amendments of 1965 took place (amendments to the 1944 Public Health Service Act), the final bill bore little resemblance to the original recommendations. An avalanche of revisions had been presented to appease special interest groups. Most disappointing for Mary and the citizen lobbyists was that the categorical research targets were blurred.

"The intention was to attack these major diseases," she said a few months later. "[They were] cut of course by the National Institutes of Health leadership, in the form of Dr. Shannon and some others. They loathe having any specifics attached to anything that they're doing." She reiterated her assertion that "they're fearful that nothing will result, and they don't want to be put on the spot to do something that they're not at all sure they can accomplish."

Mary was one of the nearly 250 people who were at the bill's East Room signing, many of whom had originally been opposed to the idea of the commission. But there they were, happily taking pens and shaking hands with the president. Still, working with LBJ from the commission's conception to this legislation had only served to confirm Mary's opinion of him. He was a man with a noble spirit. He had a sympathetic comprehension of human problems, realizing full well that if health crises were happening to him, they were happening to tens of millions of other people, too. This president had just done more for the welfare of his fellow Americans in two years than had any other president before him in the 189-year history of the nation. And that gave Mary great satisfaction.

Chapter 10

~

"A Disaster of Such
Unparalleled Proportion"

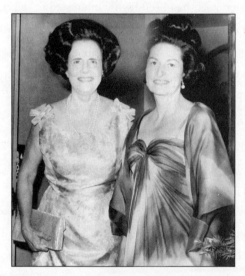

Mary and Lady Bird Johnson at a party at
Mary's Beekman Place home, June 2, 1966.

I t could have ended there, in 1965. With the signing of the Heart Disease,
Cancer, and Stroke Amendments, Mary could have rested on her laurels,
having so much else to fill her life: fabulous homes, fabulous trips, fabulous
art, fabulous parties. Her detractors were certain her motivation for such tireless
lobbying could only be fame and fortune (she already had plenty of both) or that
she was seeking power and praise (she was regularly recognized with plaudits
and awards). Few could believe she simply wanted to relieve suffering and better

lives. She would later say, "I think sometimes we might have been less resented if we'd been less successful." But that wasn't her style.

As 1966 unfolded, the public focus of the DeBakey commission's thirty-five recommendations narrowed to just one: the Regional Medical Programs. It was an exciting project, to be sure, but it prompted questions. Did the responsibility for a given region's RMP rest with the health leadership of that region? And were the development and operation of the programs meant to address the needs and capabilities of just that area? Furthermore, how long would it take funding to reach each locale? Medical professionals and medical administrators from coast to coast were unclear how to interpret it all.

The commission itself had been highly interested in the clinical drug trials that were another of their recommendations, but those never played out. Neither did the money materialize as they had envisioned. Cancer funds, for example, were cut down to just 8 percent of the total RMP budget. Most distressing of all to Mary, the RMP was originally supposed to be its own entity under the Public Health Service. Instead, it was folded into NIH as a division, to be directed by Dr. Robert Q. Marston, then associate NIH director. Although Mary thought he was a nice man, her feeling was that with RMP as a separate entity, research results would happen faster. And speed was what she was after. Americans were dying. "The NIH people in charge were non-clinicians and *not* motivated," she fumed. And she began to rethink the confidence she had placed in the organization two decades earlier.

Mary hoped Johnson would speak to these issues in his 1966 State of the Union address. It was again to be broadcast live on television, on the evening of January 12, and for the first time, it would be in color. After a cordial introduction, each of the first nine paragraphs of the president's 5,561-word address began with "I recommend." He used the word "health" five times, including, "I recommend that you [the Congress] provide the resources to carry forward, with full vigor, the great health and education programs that you enacted into law last year."[1] But there was no mention of the three killer diseases, medical research, or NIH.

Johnson uttered "Vietnam," however, thirty-four times; it was the focus of more than a third of the total speech. And just as a parent might inform their children in mid-December that there was only enough money for one of them to receive a Christmas gift, LBJ told the nation, "Because of Vietnam we cannot do all that we should, or all that we would like to do."

And then came the specifics. "While special Vietnam expenditures for the next fiscal year are estimated to increase by $5.8 billion, I can tell you that all the other expenditures put together in the entire federal budget will rise this coming year by only $0.6 billion." That translates into just $600 million, but sounded like more when attached to the word "billion." How very disappointing to the citizen lobbyists. That amount would be divided among all the nation's needs. Even if some of it actually trickled down to medical research, it would do nothing to eliminate the major diseases.

Johnson went on to explain the rationale behind America's presence in Southeast Asia: "Despite our desire to limit conflict, it was necessary to act: to hold back the mounting aggression, to give courage to the people of the South, and to make our firmness clear to the North. Thus, we began limited air action against military targets in North Vietnam. We increased our fighting force to its present strength tonight of 190,000 men." (That number would rise to over 385,000 by year's end.)[2] It appeared that the president who had declared a "war on poverty" and who the newspapers claimed had declared "war on cancer, heart disease and stroke" was now embroiled in a military war that was sucking the life out of the other, metaphorical wars. As hemlines went up—hitting mid-thigh that year—support for the Vietnam War went down. Anti-war protests, some violent, erupted from coast to coast. Johnson had additional pressures, too, in the form of the race riots occurring across the country.

The dark skies lifted slightly for the president on April 8. Just before he left Washington to spend the Easter weekend on his Texas ranch, the Albert and Mary Lasker Foundation presented him with a special award for "outstanding contributions to the health of the American people." Dr. DeBakey made the presentation in the Cabinet Room, with Mary looking on. It was lovely and meaningful, and she hoped it would remind LBJ of his commitment to medical research. But it could not mask the dismal national landscape. The next day, a U.S. military spokesman reported that 1,361 U.S. servicemen had been killed just in the month of April, compared to the 1,342 who had died in all of 1965. The war in Vietnam was stopping progress on the other war front; cancer was killing an American every two minutes.[3]

⌒

When Lady Bird Johnson first met Mary during LBJ's Senate days, she thought perhaps Mary was using her as a conduit to achieve legislative goals. Lady Bird didn't mind; she knew that was how the game was played. But the fact of the matter was that Mary genuinely liked Lady Bird. The feeling was mutual, and it wasn't long before a sincere friendship blossomed. It had become evident right after Johnson's election. Once the two women had hammered out the inauguration details together, Mary began sending Lady Bird memos with other ideas.

"Urge large-scale plantings on federal highways of native flowering trees and shrubs," one memo read, "as many states have not used their allotments under the Federal bill for planting on their highways." Mary knew that Lady Bird had the same affinity for natural beauty as she did. "Urge better lighting and lighting fixtures on highways," another memo prompted. "Stimulate national parks to improve appearance and design of motels."

"Oh, I like the idea about the highways," Lady Bird told Mary. "We have planting of highways in Texas. Wildflowers have been planted by women's clubs, and the bluebonnets look so beautiful in good years, when there's rain." Then she added, "I've appreciated so much the plantings in New York which I understand you did." Why not put together a nationwide effort, Mary suggested. But Lady Bird preferred starting small, by planting flowers in her current "hometown": Washington, D.C. She later shared that the beautification effort began "with the hope that it would have a ripple effect across the land. Everybody . . . loves his hometown."[4] The president had mentioned the program in his State of the Union address the year before. And the beautification of America officially began.

Lady Bird's first step was to invite Mary to speak at her February 5, 1965, "Women-Doers" luncheon. She had initiated the luncheons the year before to spotlight the work of American women. The informal gatherings were set up so the featured speakers were able to make their remarks seated at their tables, thus alleviating any discomfort they might have about public speaking.[5] Given Mary's aversion to being in the spotlight, that suited her perfectly. She actually did a masterly job, sharing photographs of the plantings along Park and Fifth Avenues and at the United Nations, using them as examples of what could be done. Two weeks later, Lady Bird convened the first meeting of her Committee for a More Beautiful Capital. Joining her as committee co-chair was Interior Secretary Stewart Udall. Mary was one of the twenty-two committee members present, as was Marjorie Merriweather Post (philanthropist, owner of General Foods, and owner of the Palm Beach mansion she named Mar-a-Lago). Also there was the inimitable Katharine Graham, owner of the *Washington Post*.

Washington, D.C., had become dilapidated, with poverty and racial tensions eating away at the city's neighborhoods. Lady Bird hoped the committee would undertake improvements that would help the local population. Mary knew from her experience in New York that their efforts would, without a doubt, attract tourists as well. Lady Bird envisioned making "a showcase of beauty on the Mall, which would be *used* by the American people, instead of just *looked* at."[6] To get the ball rolling, Mary donated thousands of dollars specifically for it and other tourist areas. Her money went to 9,300 azalea bushes to be planted along Pennsylvania Avenue, 200,000 daffodil bulbs added to the plantings in Rock Creek Park and along West Potomac Parkway, and 1,800 Yoshino cherry trees for planting at Hains Point. Previously barren of trees, this area, at the southern tip of East Potomac Park, would become a mass of pink blossoms every spring. Lady Bird's affection for Mary was explained in a diary entry. "In a nutshell, her [Mary's] program is, 'masses of flowers where masses pass.' Water, lights and color-mass of flowers: those things spell beautification to her."[7]

It wasn't all work and no play, however. In June of the next year, Mary gave a party for Lady Bird, who was in New York on a shopping trip with Luci and Lynda. Along with the female members of the First Family, Mary invited people "from all layers of life," as she recalled. Among the one hundred guests were Dr. Michael DeBakey, Laurance Rockefeller and his wife (he was the grandson of Standard oil co-founder John D. Rockefeller), Katharine Graham, Arthur Sulzberger (publisher of the *New York Times*), Leonard Goldberg (head of the American Broadcasting Company), and Angela Lansbury (in town as the lead in *Mame* on Broadway). It was done in Mary's classic, multipurpose entertaining style. First and foremost, her parties were always fun. And bringing together powerful and popular individuals not only made for a great party but also allowed guests to mingle with people they might otherwise not have known. Mary would, of course, be remembered for providing that opportunity. And she would cash in that IOU whenever the crusade needed it.

The evening was lovely, with clear skies and temperatures in the high sixties. Dutch Adler's band was playing on the second floor of the Beekman Place house, and as the guests danced the twist, the room got hot. Windows were thrown open and the party continued in high spirits until the doorbell rang at 1:05 a.m. Two officers from New York's Seventeenth Precinct had come about a noise complaint. In shock, Mary promised to shut the windows immediately. Fortunately, Lady Bird and Luci had left ten minutes earlier. But Lynda, who had arrived late, was still there and helped close the offending windows, drawing the drapes tightly over them.

When one entertains at that level, with the First Lady among the revelers, word of the police arriving is big news. The next day, the incident was discussed on radio and television, while newspapers from New York to Tacoma and from London to Cape Town carried the story. Mary was mortified. LBJ, however, took it all in stride. At the President's Ball a few weeks later, he told reporters, "Mrs. Johnson says we'll be okay tonight if we leave here by midnight!"[8]

A little over a week after the party, on June 11, Johnson was in New York to attend a President's Club dinner at the Waldorf Astoria. With membership fees at $1,000, those who belonged to the club and could pay to attend the functions could also afford a donation to the Democratic Party, which was the purpose of the event. Mary sat next to LBJ at dinner and shared her frustrations with him about the RMP. She stressed that no other program in the history of the country had ever focused on the diseases that cause 71 percent of the nation's deaths. "The minute that antibiotics cleared the infections up," Mary explained, "and the drugs against TB cleared that away, and the fear of polio was eliminated by vaccines, there was a hiatus. Nobody moved to say 'What's next?'" She finished with a bang. "*These* things are next!"

Mary told Johnson that she felt the commission's recommendations had been horribly watered down. She shared, too, the chronic struggle to increase research funds. "Give me a memo," he told her. In four days, she hand-delivered it to him in the Oval Office, and immediately went into great detail about the critical need for more money in the budget for NIH.

"Vietnam is going badly," Johnson explained. "We're spending a lot for the war effort, and now here you are, putting me under so much pressure for more money we haven't got." She began spouting figures again until he agreed to take action.

Two weeks later, Johnson called a White House meeting, inviting all the NIH directors, the surgeon general (now Dr. William Stewart), and John Gardner, secretary of the Department of Health, Education, and Welfare. The topic of the day was how to transform research results into answers to the problem of the three killers. Johnson emphatically explained to reporters that he had assembled this "strategy council in the war against disease" to begin a review of the "targets and the timetable they have set for winning this war." But he also underscored that it appeared "too much energy was being spent on basic research" and not enough was being spent on something tangible to help the population.[9] Having had no warning why LBJ had called the meeting, everyone in the room was shaken. They also seethed beneath the surface, knowing the source of his words. Mary Lasker had just gotten the president (who they knew "wasn't sophisticated enough to understand research") to bring down the hammer.[10]

The "strategy council" went to work and presented the president with a five-hundred-page report early in 1967. It's not certain that he read the entire report. However, it was important, Mary told Johnson, for him to meet with the group again, to show that his interest was genuine. She had hoped his tone toward them would be similar to that of the previous meeting. But LBJ took a different approach. Helicoptering the nine miles from Washington to the NIH campus in Bethesda, he called it "the world's largest medical research complex" and a "one billion dollar success story," in reference to their nearly $1 billion budget.[11] There was no hammer this time, just platitudes.

Mary knew that presidents were pulled in a thousand directions. She was doubtful that LBJ's visit had done anything to speed up research. Still, maintaining the best possible working relationships with government officials was crucial. Given all else Johnson had to cope with, there just wasn't enough time or energy for him to force NIH to be more goal-oriented. It was disappointing.

Two years earlier, when the commission made its report, DeBakey had written a cover letter to the president. In it, he had included words from famed engineer Charles F. Kettering: "No disease is incurable; it only seems so because of the ignorance of man." Mary reread those words, and on a whim she found a copy of the 1937 act that created NIH. Its purpose, she read, was to make grants to study disease. Glaringly absent was any specific language about eliminating, treating, or controlling those diseases. Those opposing concepts were the very definitions of basic and applied research, respectively. She was thunderstruck: the NIH directors were actually doing the job the act spelled out.

"Congress had assumed that it was implicit," Mary later explained. "If you established a Cancer Institute, it meant you were against cancer, and were going to plan to eliminate it." She assumed full responsibility for having furthered this enormous error. Using language similar to that in the original bill, she had, more or less, written the National Heart Act (which created the Heart Institute), and then she used that model to create the other institutes. How could she have been so obtuse? Only a change in the language laying out the purpose of all the institutes could achieve her goals. And that would be a monstrously large task, if it was even possible.

Mary was far too hard on herself. When she and Florence had begun their lobbying in 1944, NIH was just a single institute, with NCI existing as an appendage. Now NCI was a full-fledged institute itself, joining institutes devoted to mental health, the heart, dental and craniofacial research, arthritis and metabolic diseases, diabetes/digestive/kidney diseases, and child health and human development. What had formerly been called the Microbiology Institute had been reimagined as the Institute of Allergy and Infectious Diseases, and rightly so, given the structure of NIH. As one legislator had put it, "Who ever died of microbiology?"

While Mary may not have been an active participant in the creation of all nine institutes, her work certainly paved the way for the birth of many. And that was a tremendous achievement. Yet, of all the diseases and conditions the institutes addressed, cancer was still the disease most prevalent in Mary's mind. Albert's death fifteen years earlier might have contributed to her feelings. Maybe it was the disease's enigmatic nature, almost as if it refused to be conquered. Thrown into that mix was surely her frustration at the glacial pace of research. Scientists looked at disease as a problem to be solved. Mary looked at it as an enemy.

Mary's friend Truman Capote had been writing short stories and novels for twenty years, including *Breakfast at Tiffany's*. But Capote's fame was sealed when *In Cold Blood*, his "non-fiction novel," as he described it, hit the market in January 1966. The book detailed the horrific and seemingly inexplicable murders of four members of the Clutter family in western Kansas. It was an overnight success, earning Capote $2 million in just the first year (nearly $18 million today).[12] And success like that was the perfect reason to throw a party.

What evolved, however, wasn't just a party. Over the years, the quirky Capote had carefully cultivated relationships with politicians, celebrities, and members of high society, which was how he knew Mary. Her name was among the 540 who received invitations to what he called his "dance." Others dubbed it a ball, but those who referred to it as the "Decadent Party of the Decade" were more accurate.[13]

The November 28 event was held in the four-thousand-square-foot white-and-gold Grand Ballroom of the Plaza Hotel, which would be splashed with red decor and candlelit for the occasion. Guests were instructed to wear white or black and, for maximum intrigue and glamour, were to be masked.[14] "This sounded like an unusual effort on the part of people who are used to going to parties in fairly routine evening clothes," Mary later chuckled. "It excited the most enormous amount of talk. Mrs. Rose Kennedy had her secretary call to ask me what was I going to do. [There was] great consultation among the ladies as to how to dress, how to have masks made, and this and that."

In the end, Rose Kennedy wore a white gown with a gold embroidered cape, while Mary was in a silver and white dress, with a white satin mask, carrying a fan of white feathers. The ball itself didn't begin until ten, but Capote had issued other plans for the hours before the ball. Sixteen private dinner parties were to be held throughout the city for the most celebrated of his invitees. He hand-selected the hosts and hostesses, and then gave them each his prearranged guest lists. Mary was to dine at William and Babe Paley's home. She sat between Gloria Guinness (wife of Loel Guinness, of brewery fame) and Marella Agnelli (wife of Gianni Agnelli, president and principal shareholder of Fiat).

Guests of this caliber were accustomed to paying top dollar for a gala, and then expected to pay more in the way of donations. But as one pre-event newspaper piece explained, "There's no charity involved, no benefit, no cause . . . it's just for fun and Truman's paying for it." Indeed he did, to the tune of $16,000 (the equivalent of nearly $143,000, $264 per person) today.

The anticipation of the guests was matched by that of the press. "I've never seen a party so publicized in my lifetime!" Mary laughed. That kind of publicity brought throngs of celebrity watchers and cameramen, who braved the relentless, cold rain as they awaited the arrival of the guests. Capote had hired five security men and two secretaries to check invitations and to keep gate-crashers out. "The costumes and get-ups were fascinating," Mary later marveled. "And then the great mixtures of people!"

Capote had selected his close friend Katharine Graham as the guest of honor, a thank-you for feting him after the publication of *In Cold Blood*. They posted themselves in the foyer, welcoming the endless tsunami of personalities, which included many of the Kennedy clan (Rose, Jackie, Jackie's sister Lee Radziwill, and JFK's sisters and their husbands), Lynda Bird Johnson, Margaret

Truman, actresses Lauren Bacall and Tallulah Bankhead, Frank Sinatra (with his young wife Mia Farrow), a slew of politicians and titans of industry, and everyone from Kansas whom Capote had interviewed for his book (minus the now-executed killers).

"Truman himself was so well masked," Mary later related, "that when I came into the party, someone shook my hand very cordially. Naturally I shook it back, but didn't realize who it was." Despite his elaborate costume instructions for guests, Capote's mask had set him back 35¢ at the famed toy store F. A. O. Schwarz.

The throngs danced alternately to the popular Peter Duchin and his orchestra and then to the Soul Brothers, a rock-and-roll group. They wandered from one informal table to another, gulped hundreds of bottles of Taittinger champagne, and unmasked at midnight to graze at the buffet of chicken in wine sauce, spaghetti à la Bolognese, scrambled eggs, bacon, and sausages. The music didn't stop till eight the next morning, although Mary had called it quits at one-thirty. Capote's ball had provided quite a diversion from the year's earlier frustrations. But there were more on the horizon.

⟿

On Tuesday morning, January 10, 1967, Representative John Fogarty arrived at the Longworth Office Building on Independence Avenue in Washington. It was a mild day, in the low forties, with a winter sun darting in and out of the clouds. Fogarty would be sworn in for his fourteenth term when the Ninetieth Congress was called to order in a few hours. But at eight-thirty, as he made his way to his office, the building's halls were nearly empty. When the congressman's aide arrived at nine-fifty, he found Fogarty's dead body.[15]

The fifty-three-year-old's death sent shock waves through the capital city and beyond. "Mr. Public Health"—an often-used moniker—had died of a heart attack. Ironically, a year earlier, President Johnson had awarded him the Heart of the Year Award. In his remarks that day, the president had said, "The International Health Act of 1966 is to launch a cooperative effort by all of the world's people to make a determined and organized attempt to conquer disease wherever it exists in human beings. . . . The world cannot wait. The clock is ticking."[16]

No one could have known that Fogarty would run out of time so soon. Mary had once said of him that his work in Congress on behalf of the crusade added "to the average length of life of people all over the world. He's basically and deeply a humanitarian." Fogarty had played his part well in the annual medical research budget dance. Whenever the executive branch submitted its figures, the amount for NIH was always lower than asked for. Fogarty would berate the White House for its cutbacks, interviewing NIH officials and crusade-supplied citizen witnesses to support the original ask. He would raise the appropriations amount and submit a Gorman-written report. Mary would miss him greatly.

Senator Hill would miss Fogarty, too. His part in the dance had been to raise Fogarty's NIH budget amounts even more in the Senate. Now, Hill's counterpart on the House appropriations subcommittee would be Daniel Flood, a Pennsylvanian whose waxed mustache made people see him as a combination of Salvador Dalí and the cartoon villain who ties the innocent victim to the train tracks. Flood had been diagnosed with esophageal cancer in the early 1960s and miraculously survived, but it hadn't softened his heart toward the crusade. "You would think because he was a victim of cancer of the esophagus he would be more interested in medical research," Mary observed, "but the truth is that it's the opposite."

The year would not get better. As the Summer of Love began, turmoil spilled out across the country. Race riots ripped cities apart, the worst occurring in Detroit, leaving it a burning battlefield. President Johnson sent in the army to restore order. By the time it was over, forty people had died, two thousand more were injured, and five thousand were left homeless. Equally tragic was the conflict in Southeast Asia. For the first time in history, Americans at home were being given a ringside seat to war. Footage of the day's battles in Vietnam—mud and explosions, body bags and fear—streamed into living rooms every night on the news broadcasts of all three networks. Five hundred soldiers were dying each month, and Americans were getting angry about it. Those of the younger generation who weren't drafted watched their buddies being sent in. Many wanted no part of it, marching in anti-establishment, anti-government, anti-war protests.

The year ended with an aggravation dumped directly in Mary's lap. The December issue of *Atlantic Monthly* featured an article written by Elizabeth Drew. Entitled "The Health Syndicate," Drew outlined the efforts of the crusaders to increase research funding. Mary described it as "really unfriendly and scurrilous." She also felt she'd been duped. "I spoke to the author on the telephone once. She said she wanted my opinion of the research policies of the PHS, or something like that." Drew had given no indication of the gist of her article. Then Drew spoke to Mike Gorman, who, Mary said, "thought she was sympathetic and he was giving her background material. He had no idea that she was going to quote him verbatim, which she did largely." Unfortunately, the verbatim segments that made it into print were not flattering.

Mary consulted her lawyer: "Listen, this is character assassination, and I'd like to sue *Atlantic Monthly*." Her lawyer calmly told her it would be a mistake. Still, Mary insisted, there were two really unforgivable offenses. The first was in regard to Mary's personal life. "She was misinformed about things, especially the extent of my husband's wealth, which is very embarrassing . . . to be thought much richer than one is." (The article reported that Mary was worth more than $80 million.) But it was the second offense that really galled her.

"The main premise—the most damaging thing about it—was that cancer, heart and stroke only affected older people, so did it [research] really matter? Everybody is going to die anyway, why not let them die?" Mary went on angrily. "Now, the truth is that cancer and heart are the major causes of death from the age of one to twenty, and twenty to forty, as well as from forty on. So all the criticism and snide attitude is really vitiated by the fact that she didn't know her figures. And most readers wouldn't know the figures, either. It was damaging."

If being passionate about a cause was a crime, Mary and her fellow citizen lobbyists were certainly guilty. Likewise, if being persistent toward achieving a goal is also a crime, that would have garnered a second guilty verdict. However, the lives saved by the research they lobbied for were never brought to light. It would have been ample pardon for their crimes.

⚊

New York City welcomed 1968 with four inches of snow and single-digit temperatures. In retrospect, it was an omen for what became an annus horribilis. On January 20, Lister Hill announced he would retire from the Senate after his current term ended the following year. The seventy-three-year-old had spent nearly half a century in Congress, fifteen years in the House and thirty in the Senate. His motivation for retirement was concern for his beloved wife, Henrietta, who suffered from Parkinson's disease. Mary knew the challenges that awaited the crusade without Hill, having just gone through them in the House after Fogarty's death. But she was also very sympathetic to Henrietta's condition. Ever the health connector, she told the Hills about a newly approved drug that had shown wonderful promise in Parkinson's treatment. Once Henrietta was on it, her condition vastly improved, but the senator's decision was final.

Eleven days later, Vietnam celebrated Tet, the Lunar New Year festival. The Viet Cong used the holiday to launch a stunning series of orchestrated attacks against key cities in South Vietnam. It came to be known as the Tet Offensive, lasting until March 28. Johnson had already lied repeatedly about America's military progress, and he continued the practice in his statements about the Tet Offensive, assuring America that victory was just around the corner. In reality, 1968 would become the deadliest year of the war: a total of 16,592 Americans perished.

As fatalities mounted, the president announced he would address the nation at nine o'clock on the night of Sunday, March 31, to explain troop deployments and military strategy. Gripped with anxiety, insecurity, and a multitude of pressures, the fifty-nine-year-old Johnson looked haggard when he began to speak. After thirty-nine minutes of discussing the war, including to say that he was partially halting the U.S. bombing, he dropped a bombshell of his own in the last minute of his speech: "I shall not seek, and I will not accept the nomination of my party for another term as your president."[17]

Across America, jaws dropped. Only a very small circle had known it was coming, including Lady Bird, the couple's daughters, Vice President Humphrey, Horace Busby (LBJ's speechwriter and one of his closest confidants), and the typist who put that portion of the speech into the teleprompter just minutes before LBJ went on the air.[18] Mary watched from her Palm Springs vacation spot and was as stunned as the rest of the country. She caught her breath and phoned the White House, where the switchboard was already on fire with incoming calls. When she finally did get through, it was to speak to a very calm Lady Bird. Mary realized that she and LBJ had come to the decision together. After much time considering the pros and cons, it was the right thing for their future.

The next morning, newspapers were full of the implications that the president's declaration had unleashed. "Rarely in American history have political events careened over so wayward a course as they have in recent weeks," declared one. Johnson's surprise announcement, it went on, "created a minor trauma in the ranks of both Democrats and Republicans."[19] On the Democratic side, Minnesota senator Eugene McCarthy had been planning a run as the anti-war candidate against the assumed incumbent. Senator Robert Kennedy, too, had planned to be a candidate, also anti-war, and running on a racial and economic justice platform. A week after Johnson's speech, Humphrey threw his hat into the ring.

In the Republican camp, Richard Nixon was a strong favorite, followed by former New York governor Nelson Rockefeller and former California governor and actor Ronald Reagan. Nixon and his team had been working on chipping away at the Johnson administration's track record, believing, as everyone had, that he would be the Democratic nominee. With LBJ out of the race, new strategies had to be devised. But more shocks were in store for the country.

Five days after the bombshell speech, and in an already racially charged national atmosphere, Dr. Martin Luther King Jr. was shot as he stood on the balcony of a Memphis, Tennessee, motel. He died an hour later. Two months after that, on June 5, Robert Kennedy was celebrating his victory in the California primary at a rally at the Ambassador Hotel in Los Angeles. As he exited through the hotel kitchen, he, too, was shot, and died twenty-six hours afterward. That murder made Hubert Humphrey the clear Democratic front-runner.

Mary had long been a close friend of Humphrey's, financially supporting his campaigns. She related, "The last time I saw Humphrey, he said, 'If I'm elected, you'll have everything you want, Mary.' He's really interested in health problems because he was a pharmacist, and he's had severe problems in his own family."

The Republican convention was held in early August in Miami Beach. For the fourth time, Nixon was nominated on the Republican ticket (twice previously as Eisenhower's vice president and then as president in 1960). Later in the month, the Democratic convention was held in Chicago. It was rife with drama, as city police officers beat anti-war protesters outside the convention hall, with the violence playing out live on television. The nomination, however, was less dramatic, with Humphrey selected on the first round of balloting.

Mary was asked her opinion of a possible Nixon presidency. Her answer: "I think the prospects for getting anything much done are very poor because Nixon has never said anything about health or medical research." It had been eight years since she had described the notion of Nixon in the White House as a potential "disaster of such unparalleled proportion."

Election day was Tuesday, November 5, but the vote counting went on until the early hours of Wednesday morning. In the end, the "disaster" became a reality. Humphrey lost the popular vote by just 0.7 percent but took only 35.5 percent of the Electoral College. Richard Milhous Nixon became the thirty-seventh president of the United States. And like Kennedy and Johnson before him, he was about to wade into the same two wars: Vietnam and cancer.

Chapter 11

⟜

"A Simple Pill That a Simple Physician Can Give to a Suffering Patient"

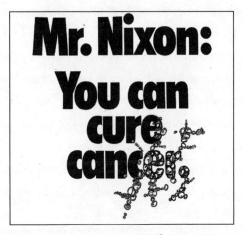

*"Mr. Nixon" ad created by the Citizens Committee
for the Conquest of Cancer, circa 1969.*

"We cannot learn from one another until we stop shouting at one another—until we speak quietly enough so that our words can be heard as well as our voices."[1] Newly sworn in President Nixon stood on the steps of the Capitol's East Portico, speaking words of hope and healing to a divided nation. The forty-degree temperatures were mild for January 20, although rain was predicted. It was, perhaps, an omen of the cloud under which this president would begin his administration. Not far from the Capitol, anti-war protests were heating up. Rocks and beer cans would later be hurled at the president's limousine during the inaugural parade.

The Nixons had begun their day with a nine-thirty prayer breakfast at the State Department, and then traveled to the White House for a quick meeting with the Johnsons. LBJ's term would officially end at noon, when the swearing-in ceremony began.[2] But before he closed the book on his presidency, Johnson carried out one more official act, awarding Mary the Medal of Freedom, the highest civilian honor a chief executive can bestow. There was no ceremony, as Mary was not in Washington, obviously not going to the inaugural ball. So a friendly telephone chat and kind words sufficed. The medal's accompanying citation reiterated LBJ's sentiments: "Mary Lasker has inspired understanding and productive legislation. . . . In medical research, in adding grace and beauty to the environment, and in exhorting her fellow citizens to rally to the cause of progress, she has made a lasting imprint on the quality of life in this country." Of course, neither Mary nor the president could know for certain the crusade's future. But with the Republicans' history of slashing health budgets, she stood at the foot of a very tall mountain.

At least the annus horribilis was over, and it had included one welcome change. On August 31, 1968, having reached the statutory retirement age, director James Shannon left NIH. Replacing him was Robert Q. Marston, who had been at NIH in the early fifties, left for academia, and then returned in 1966 as director of the RMP.

"I'm very glad we got Shannon out," Mary said of the man who had blocked the crusade for so long. "At least with Marston, or anybody else in the job, we have a chance to get more clinical research approved of." Her enthusiasm for the new director, however, was lukewarm. "Marston is a very nice man from Mississippi. . . . But he's a man who is not at all driving. He's an ameliorator."

She and Hill had suggested other, more aggressive candidates to HEW secretary Wilbur Cohen, but Marston was the only one they could all agree upon. Maybe the new blood would provide a new direction. After all their work to get the 1965 amendment passed, its disappointing focus was now only on supplying health services. While that was an admirable task, it completely obfuscated all of the other recommendations, including research. Mary had feared it would eventually happen as soon as she saw the bill's final language. Carleton B. Chapman, dean of the Dartmouth Medical School, had seen it too, remarking, "Its [the amendment's] primary emphasis [is] on regionalization of the nation's health service rather than on conquering killer diseases."[3] A *Boston Globe* medical writer left the idea of medical research out of the picture completely when he wrote, "Regional Medical Programs are founded on the premise that local talent with Federal funding can find local answers to the problems of how to provide quality health care to all citizens."[4]

The AMA had stopped fighting federally funded medical research (abandoning a stance that was ridiculous for an organization whose membership is sworn to heal), but they were not fooled by a writer using the terms "health care" and "federal funding" in the same sentence. It still smelled like national health insurance, and they would have none of it. Although Mary wished every citizen could receive the kind of health care she had the ability to pay for, she had come to the conclusion that she would do best to focus her energies in one direction, one that would *not* be impeded by the AMA. In the new administration's first year, two-thirds of all people diagnosed with cancer would die of their disease. The only answer was applied medical research, bringing new discoveries to patients who needed them. She was hoping for "a simple pill that a simple physician can give to a suffering patient." Could Nixon be the president to make that a reality?

⟿

The night that Mary first met Adlai Stevenson in 1952, he was in the company of the darkly handsome William McCormick Blair Jr., then thirty-six years old. Bill's mother was part of the illustrious McCormick family; a great-great-uncle had modernized farming by inventing the McCormick reaper. His father was a wealthy Chicago financier. A lawyer by profession, Bill was a partner at the Chicago firm of Stevenson and Wirtz and was Adlai Stevenson's closest friend and most influential advisor. As Mary's friendship with Stevenson grew, so did the one she forged with Bill, who was so impressed on his first visit to her farm in Amenia that he teased her, "Mary, are you sure you're a Democrat? Most Democrats don't live like this!" That was funnier still since they were all friends of the Kennedys, who very much lived as Mary did.

In fact, it was Eunice Kennedy Shriver (JFK's sister) and her husband, Sargent, who changed Bill's life. The Shrivers lived on Chicago's North Side in a high-rise with sweeping views of Lake Michigan. In the late fifties, as JFK was preparing for his presidential run, Eunice had a dinner party, and invited Blair. She also included the newly divorced daughter of a neighbor, twenty-eight-year-old Catherine Gerlach. Everyone called her Deeda, a name her brother had created when she was born, as he was unable to pronounce "Catherine." Like Bill (now forty-three), Deeda, too, had grown up in Chicago society. She was as beautiful as he was handsome, and it wasn't long before a romance blossomed.

One month after President Kennedy had selected Bill to be the ambassador to Denmark, in March 1961, he and Deeda announced their engagement. By this time, Mary had come to love the exquisitely stylish young woman as much as the future groom did. Their fairytale wedding took place on September 9, in the seventeenth-century Frederiksborg Castle, twenty-two miles from Copenhagen. The scene at the former home to Danish kings was best described by a *Chicago Tribune* writer: "At 4:10 pm, the sun, hidden so much lately, broke through in full glory just as the bride, in a Balenciaga wedding gown of ice blue French gauze, crossed the cobblestone courtyard and entered the chapel. . . . On her dark hair was a blue froth of veil embroidered with fragile blue flowers."[5]

The five hundred guests included Rose Kennedy, Eunice and Sargent Shriver, Anna Rosenberg, and, of course, Mary, who was already in Europe at La Fiorentina. The Blairs' European honeymoon would include a stopover at Mary's villa. When Johnson became president, he appointed Bill as ambassador to the Philippines. Once that stint was completed in 1968, the couple and their six-year-old son moved to Washington, and Robert Kennedy asked Bill to become the first director of the Kennedy Center for the Performing Arts (which would open in 1971 under Blair's direction).

The hours in Deeda's days, however, had long before been determined. Shortly after the Blairs' wedding, she had become Mary's protégé. Whenever she visited New York, she stayed at Beekman Place. After Deeda mentioned she had not been allowed to study biology during her twelve years at Sacred Heart School, Mary took her to meet Dr. David Karnofsky of Memorial Sloan Kettering. The famed chemotherapy researcher allowed Deeda to shadow him everywhere. "It was the most extraordinary learning experience," she later recalled. And once the Blairs returned to the States, Mary invited Deeda to be vice president of the Lasker Foundation.

Like Mary, Deeda was able to blend a love of style and beautiful things with an ardor for fighting ugly disease and bettering the human condition. After all, as a journalist friend of Deeda's wisely observed, "the word 'elegant' is in regular use in both fashion and science."[6] Since Florence Mahoney had become even more focused on mental health and was now further occupied as a board member of Eunice Shriver's National Institute of Child Health and Human Development, Deeda stepped in to fill the gap. And despite their thirty-two-year age difference, the two women became very close.

Deeda was, Mary said, "one of the great joys of my life." Sometimes with Bill, sometimes alone, Deeda spent several weeks every summer with Mary in France. They traveled to Paris and stayed at the Ritz, attending the couture shows. But the five-hundred-mile train ride to and from La Fiorentina gave them ample time to pore over scientific journals and Mary's now massive article files.

Deeda greatly admired Mary's ability to bring people with power together, entertaining actress Greta Garbo, Princess Grace of Monaco, and Michael DeBakey all at the same dinner party. That tradition would receive an enormous injection stateside at the Blairs' newly purchased 6,200-square-foot brick Georgian mansion. Just five minutes from Georgetown, its nearly one and a half acres sat on a woodsy ravine on Foxhall Road. Deeda had wanted her house to be "the most tranquil of retreats."[7] Its multiple levels made it perfect for entertaining and, more importantly, an epicenter for medical research lobbying.

⁓

As those in the crusade had expected, Nixon lowered LBJ's NIH budget almost immediately upon taking office. The Democrats, however, still maintained their majority in both chambers of Congress. Mary felt the first hearings intended to ramp the NIH coffers back up—which took place in May 1969—went fairly well, with Farber, DeBakey, and others testifying as to the need. But she never took anything for granted, so she and Deeda organized a dinner at the Blairs' home in honor of former vice president Hubert Humphrey.

Mother Nature provided a lovely evening for the June 11 party, the threat of rain showers never materializing. Guests were ushered from the marble-paved entry into the drawing room for cocktails and hors d'oeuvres. Besides the guest of honor, they had invited Democratic representatives Robert Casey and George Mahon of Texas, Daniel Flood of Pennsylvania (chair of the health appropriations subcommittee), William Hull of Missouri, Neal Smith of Iowa, and their respective wives. Dinner was served in the dining room, and both it and the accompanying conversation were lovely.

Over the next days, Mary went to collect her reward for being co-hostess: the congressmen's assurances of financial support for medical research. To her dismay, all of them were disinterested and vague. She recalled, "Mahon, chairman of the full Appropriations Committee, had a brother dying of lung cancer. I went to see him, bearing some information about a new drug that might be helpful for lung cancer. He was unsympathetic to any raise in research figures, cancer or any other."

Mahon had even bragged to her that he had appointed his particular committee members because they would be against additional funds for research. Indeed they were, and they voted for the Nixon budget without a whimper. It was time to create a new legislative army in the House. The Senate looked a little rosier. Lister Hill's replacement as chair of the Labor and Public Welfare Committee was Texan Ralph Yarborough. Known as "Smilin' Ralph," he had entered the Senate in 1957 (the year LBJ became majority leader) and used the same cornpone campaign slogan throughout his career: "Let's put the jam on the lower shelf so the little people can reach it."

Yarborough had been riding with LBJ and Lady Bird in the motorcade when President Kennedy was assassinated. He became a big supporter of his fellow Texan's Great Society, and it was through the Johnsons that Mary first got to know him. Yarborough became chair of the health subcommittee, happily assuming Hill's "Mr. Health" persona. Asked why he hadn't chosen any of the other subcommittees, he replied, "Because the great need is there."[8] But Yarborough's resumé had one item that would become the most important to Mary: in 1958 he had been on the subcommittee whose work resulted in the creation of the National Aeronautics and Space Administration (NASA).

⟿

Shortly after Alan Shepard's fifteen minutes in space in 1961, President Kennedy had told a joint session of Congress, "I believe that this nation should commit itself to achieving the goal, before this decade is out, of landing a man on the moon and returning him safely to earth."[9] Eight years later, on July 20, 1969, Neil Armstrong and Edwin "Buzz" Aldrin fulfilled that promise. After leaving their Saturn V space vehicle (Apollo 11), launched four days before from the Kennedy Space Center in Florida, they flew the lunar module, *Eagle*, to the moon's surface. Armstrong came down *Eagle*'s ladder first, at about 10:56 p.m. EST, and Aldrin followed a few minutes later.

The astronauts spent two hours and thirteen minutes on the moon's surface. They planted an American flag, took photos, and gathered twenty pounds of rock samples. They also had a chat with President Nixon. "I just can't tell you how proud we all are of what you have done," the president extolled. "For every American, this has to be the proudest day of our lives."[10]

That triumph shared newspaper headlines with another story: "Formal Charges Filed Against Kennedy."[11] Just twenty-four hours before the lunar landing, a car driven by Senator Ted Kennedy plunged into Poucha Pond on Chappaquiddick Island in Massachusetts. Kennedy escaped; his twenty-eight-year-old passenger, campaign worker Mary Jo Kopechne, did not. Prior to that night, it appeared that the 1972 Democratic nomination for president was Kennedy's if he wanted it. The watery accident washed away not only the hopes of that but also a great deal of the senator's credibility overall. He had left the scene, not reporting the event for nine hours, claiming shock and trauma.

At his July 25 court hearing, Kennedy pled guilty to leaving the scene of an accident and was given a two-month suspended jail sentence. Later that evening, he delivered a televised statement, again defending himself in Kopechne's death. He also offered to resign his Senate position, asking the people of Massachusetts for direction. Telephone calls and telegrams poured in, both to the newspapers and the Kennedy family itself, heavily in favor of the senator remaining in office.

Like all Americans, Mary was following both stories. The successful moon landing caused her to recall a visit she had had with President Johnson five years earlier. They were both in Palm Springs, enjoying a winter escape from the frozen East Coast. "You know, we're making big efforts in outer space," Mary told LBJ. (NASA's Project Gemini was in full swing that year.) "Why shouldn't we also make an effort in 'inner space,' meaning more medical research?"

Someone else had thought of connecting space exploration with medical exploration. Earlier in 1969 Mary had read *Cure for Cancer: A National Goal,* a book written by Colorado pharmacologist Dr. Solomon Garb, which laid out Garb's belief that the time had come to reevaluate the country's cancer research.[12] All leads, new ones as well as those already in existence, should be taken as far as possible. More money was essential, he thought, to make that happen, along with this crucial element: America should take on "a commitment to make the cure . . . of cancer a national goal in the same way that putting a man into orbit around the earth was made a national goal and then achieved." The space program, he said, had greatly benefited from living within an independent agency, reporting directly to the president.

Mary had been electrified by Garb's book. She bought copies and shared them with friends, and she invited Garb to come visit her at Beekman Place, which he happily did. They became friends, finding agreement with each other on practically everything. Garb was added to the list of congressional citizen witnesses, his enthusiastic style matching that of the others who often testified. Combining the premise of his book and the lunar landing, why not launch a moon shot for cancer? Mary was now seriously questioning whether NIH was the right agency to find an end to the disease. There were too many things impeding progress, most notably bureaucracy. But an independent, NASA-like organization whose sole focus would be to eradicate cancer forever—now, that could work.

Mary delivered a copy of *Cure for Cancer* to Senator Yarborough in June 1969. "I think you should appoint a commission to advise your committee about the legislation in connection with such an objective," she suggested to him. Then she innocently added, "The National Cancer Institute might be just one factor in it." Focusing on his role in the creation of the space agency, she thought there "might have to be a special Cancer Conquest Administration, like the NASA Administration, outside of the cancer institute to get this done."

Yarborough was interested, but overwhelmed with anxiety. He was running for another term in 1970 and was concerned about the primary he had to win first. Conservative Texas Democrats had seethed when, after Johnson announced he wouldn't run in 1968, Yarborough spoke out against the Vietnam War, supporting the liberal, anti-war Bobby Kennedy. Mary promised to help Yarborough in his campaign, as she had before, and to bring him a memo with the scope of her idea. Delivered a few weeks later, the memo was entitled "Need for a Commission on the Conquest of Cancer as a National Goal by 1976." It was filled with statistics (as her memos always were) and contained a list of twenty-six names—a combination of medical and lay individuals—that she suggested for the commission. The senator resisted, saying he was so busy, he didn't know how he'd have time to phone and persuade them all.

So Mary thought perhaps having the president involved in the commission would get it moving sooner. Since HEW was the guardian of NIH, it was time for her to meet the new Nixon team. The department's scope was broad, and its presidentially appointed leadership sometimes had connection to only one of its three areas. Nixon's choice for the department secretary, attorney Robert Finch, had no connection to any of them. He had met the president—then a freshman congressman—after World War II. Nixon had encouraged Finch to pursue a law degree, which he did, and then he became Nixon's 1960 campaign manager. After Nixon's defeat, Finch went back to California to ultimately be elected lieutenant governor under Ronald Reagan. Finch later served as Nixon's 1968 campaign manager, and after the election the president gave him carte blanche to choose a cabinet position.

Within HEW, Dr. Roger Egeberg became the assistant secretary for health and scientific affairs, having previously been dean of the University of Southern California Medical School. Mary began her commission campaign with him, inviting him to dinner at Trader Vic's in late July before she left for Europe. "We are very friendly," she explained soon after, "and I hope the friendship will be constructive." When she returned to the States, she next invited Finch to lunch, this time at her home in September. That, too, was pleasant. "Although he's not well informed in the field, and has no background in medicine at all," she explained, "he was sympathetic to it [research] because his father had died of cancer."

Mary told Finch that Senator Yarborough was interested in appointing a commission for the conquest of cancer, not just to research the disease but to find answers to it *now*. She suggested the president might like to appoint the commission, and asked Finch to speak with Nixon about it, promising to send the same memo she had given to Yarborough. Then she turned up the charm, telling him she wanted to welcome him, Egeberg, and their wives to Washington by hosting a dinner with the Blairs. Among the others ultimately joining them were Senators Warren Magnuson (now the Democratic chair of the Senate Commerce Committee), Senator Jacob Javits (a Republican to whom she had donated because he was interested in heart disease research), United Auto Workers president Walter Reuther, the three men's wives, and various doctors sympathetic to the crusade. It was Mary's classic tapestry of people, never one-sided, always welcoming.

Not long after her initial meeting with Finch, Mary received a letter from fellow Wisconsinite Melvin Laird, a Republican. During his fourteen-year stint in the House, Laird served on the Appropriations Committee, giving him an odd blend of expertise in both defense and health care matters. He often worked in concert with Fogarty and had been recognized with a 1963 Lasker Public Service Award. When Nixon was elected, Laird became secretary of defense. As he explained in his letter to Mary, he was appalled when he learned the number of military families on welfare. To discern possible solutions, he was planning precisely what she was famous for: a luncheon at the Pentagon with influential people from a broad spectrum. Would she please attend?

Since this would give her yet another opportunity to be with a member of Nixon's cabinet, Mary accepted without hesitation, and made an appointment to meet with Laird before the other guests arrived. Drawing on his experience with NIH matters, she shared her idea of making cancer a national goal. Laird liked the idea and promised to speak with both Finch and the president. The idea of Nixon appointing the commission had just become more possible. Mary knew that if it was the president's idea, and if it produced substantial recommendations that could lead to a cure, Nixon's ego wouldn't be able to resist following those recommendations, and he would put the necessary money into the budget; Magnuson would then get the Senate to go along, as would Flood on the House side.

Mary had one more Republican ace up her sleeve. Back in 1945, when she and Albert were working on their successful ACS fundraising campaign, they had persuaded businessman Eric Johnston to head it up. He was a friend of Anna's— and a Republican—who had served with her on FDR's War Manpower Commission. Johnston had brought fellow Republican Elmer Bobst to the table, and the Laskers became friendly with him. A successful pharmaceutical executive, Bobst had become beloved by Richard Nixon, who considered him "an honorary father."[13] Without a doubt, Bobst was the only mutual friend Mary and Nixon had, which would make him a perfect addition to her proposed commission.

The week before Thanksgiving, she invited Bobst, along with crusade friends Foote, Farber, and Laurance Rockefeller, to her house. Once she laid out her ideas and suggested that all four of her guests be part of the commission, they discussed next steps. The obvious one was for Bobst to bring it up with the president. Fortuitously, the Nixons were having an eighty-fifth birthday party for Bobst on December 16. Amid the celebrating, he did indeed broach the subject with Nixon, but there wasn't enough time to discuss it at any length.

The president had already heard about making the end of cancer a national goal. It had been shouted at him the week before from full-page ads in the

Washington Post, New York Times, and *New York Post.* "Mr. Nixon," the ad read in enormous letters, "you can cure cancer." A smaller font followed the attention-grabber, suggesting that while he was agonizing over the budget he should re-member the agony of the 318,000 Americans who died of cancer the previous year. The ad pointed out that the government spent more each day on the mili-tary than was spent each *year* on cancer research. The latter was also enormously outspent by space research. The war against cancer "is a war in which we lost twenty-one times more lives last year than we lost in Vietnam last year. . . . Why don't we try to conquer cancer by America's 200th birthday? What a holiday that would be!"

Conveniently placed on the page was a form asking Nixon for more cancer research funding. Readers could simply fill in their address and mail it to the White House. The Citizens Committee for the Conquest of Cancer was listed at the bottom of the page, along with Foote and Garb as co-chairs. Its address was the same as the Lasker Foundation's, at UN Plaza. Mary had quietly financed the newspaper campaign to the tune of $26,000 (close to a quarter of a million today). It was money well spent: nearly eight thousand letters poured in.

Between Finch, Egeberg, Laird, Bobst, and the ad, Nixon had to have gotten the picture. "I know you've been thinking about appointing this commission but you haven't been able to do it," Mary told Yarborough. "I have a friend who's a friend of Nixon's; maybe it would be better if the president appointed a commission."

Yarborough replied sharply that it would *not* be better. He had absolutely no faith that Nixon would ever follow recommendations or add money to the bud-get for an idea that wasn't his. The senator promised her that he would take care of it. But when the capital emptied out for the holidays on December 23, nothing had yet happened. As the year slipped to a close, Mary, never one to look back at what hadn't been achieved, donned a pink and gold evening gown and headed to a friend's annual New Year's Eve party. She was confident that the events of the 1960s were merely a preparation that would pay off in the 1970s.

Two hundred miles away, Farber sat in his home office in Boston. He, too, reflected on the passing year, writing her a letter that echoed the feelings of many. "Dear Mary: The closing hours of the Old Year are still rosy with the echoes of your remarkable statement of our goals against cancer . . . I just want to tell you again what a great privilege it has been to work under your leadership in your small army dedicated to eradicate disease. . . . The health of the world owes more to you than to any one person. Sincerely yours, Sidney."[14]

⌐

Richard Nixon was a complicated man, chased by demons of insecurity and doubt, with an abhorrence of confrontation. He was a perfectionist and a control freak in the imperfect and out-of-control nation of which he had become president. And yet, as it was with Mary's work, Nixon saw the value of having a variety of individuals in his administration. Consequently, he offered positions to some with more liberal voices: Mike Wallace, Doris Kearns, and Richard Goodwin (who would become Kearns's husband in 1975). Also on that list were civil rights leaders Whitney Young and James Farmer, as well as Democrats "Scoop" Jackson and Daniel Patrick Moynihan.[15]

Nixon really wasn't interested in domestic affairs—including anything to do with the health of the country—unless it gained him a political advantage. During the 1968 campaign, he even told journalist Theodore White, "I've always thought this country could run itself domestically without a president. You need a president for foreign policy."[16] To that end, Nixon's first months in office were spent dismantling Johnson's Great Society.

But domestic affairs couldn't be ignored. Racial divisiveness continued, as did anti-war protests. Nixon had campaigned on the promise of an end to the Vietnam War. A television campaign ad had suggested the possibility of a nuclear holocaust if America didn't triumph. It included the candidate's voice saying, "This time vote like your whole world depended on it." He had even convinced the South Vietnamese president, Nguyen Van Thieu, to continue fighting until after the election, when Nixon would be able to offer the South Vietnamese more than the Democrats had. In March 1969, when the number of Americans killed in action in Vietnam stood at 33,641, he told the country he was working toward "peace with honor."[17]

Nixon was adamant about "peace with honor," but he privately proclaimed he would *not* be the "first American President to lose a war."[18] To circumvent the latter, he ordered secret bombings of Vietnam's neutral neighbors, Laos and Cambodia, through which passed the Viet Cong's main artery for moving troops and supplies (the Ho Chi Minh Trail). The secret was discovered when a wire service reporter filed a story with the *Washington Star* stating that General John Abrams had sought permission for the secret bombing. The March 25 story could only mean there was a leak in the Pentagon.

FBI director J. Edgar Hoover told the president the only way to stop leaks was wiretapping, which Nixon later called "the ultimate weapon."[19] On May 9 another article with classified information broke, again citing anonymous Pentagon sources. Five days later, after a particularly bloody ground battle that came to be known as Hamburger Hill, Nixon went live in his first televised address about Vietnam. He said he wouldn't accept a peace that was only a disguised American defeat. But he still didn't elucidate a specific path to ending the war. In truth, he felt he had been unfairly saddled with Vietnam. Kennedy had started it. Johnson had escalated it a hundredfold. Nixon was now responsible for the 539,000 troops in-country and the more than one hundred dying each week.

Enter Ted Kennedy. Speaking from the Senate floor on May 20, he said it was "senseless and irresponsible to continue to send our young men to their deaths to capture hills and positions that have no relation to ending the military conflict."[20] For Nixon, it seemed the Kennedys would forever be a thorn in his side. *They* had grown up rich; Nixon's father was an unsuccessful lemon farmer and a dirt-poor grocer. *They* were educated at prestigious private schools and universities; Nixon went to a local college, Whittier, so he could live at home.

Nixon was convinced family patriarch Joe Kennedy had stolen the 1960 election from him with illegal voting in Texas and Illinois (where Chicago mayor Richard Daley had halted the counting around midnight to assess how many more votes might need to be added to deliver the state to JFK). Those "dirty tricks" had been committed by "the most ruthless group of political operators ever mobilized for a presidential campaign," Nixon later wrote. "From that moment on, I had the wisdom and wariness of someone who had been burned by the power of the Kennedys and their money."[21]

Bobby Kennedy, before he was assassinated, had been rough with Nixon as they both prepared for the 1968 election. Nixon referred to him as the "little son of a bitch," although both he and First Lady Pat were rocked when he was killed. It was Ted, however, who Nixon felt was particularly vindictive toward him. The fourth Kennedy son was the heir presumptive for the 1972 Democratic nomination, and Ted Kennedy as president was something Nixon found personally and politically unbearable. And then Chappaquiddick happened. Nixon couldn't believe his luck. Ted was now so tainted that the White House was out of the question.

—

The invitation's return address was 1600 Pennsylvania Avenue, Washington, D.C. Mary had received letters from that address before, but never when the White House was occupied by a Republican. Yet there it was, asking her to a dinner in celebration of the exhibition of American artist Andrew Wyeth. While her preference was for impressionist art, she was intrigued by all paintings, and she found Wyeth "an easy artist to be interested in." She gladly accepted the invitation.

The February 19, 1970, black-tie event began in the East Room, where twenty-one of Wyeth's paintings (valued at $2 million) would hang for a month-long public viewing. Wyeth would be the first artist ever honored with a special White House show. President Nixon raised his glass of champagne in a toast, proclaiming Wyeth "one of the greatest painters in the world." The party of 110 then moved on to their repast of pheasant breast and wild rice.[22]

The evening was lovely; President and Mrs. Nixon were relaxed and cordial. That gave Mary an opportunity to thank him for his recent approval of funds for NCI, although it was only a small increase. "Oh yes," Nixon told her, "Bobst has been all over me about that." He made no mention of the ads or their associated bags of mail.

Exactly one month before this delightful evening, on January 19, the second session of the Ninety-first Congress had opened. Fresh from the holiday recess—although still nervous about his May primary—Yarborough was ready to move forward with the resolution proposing Mary's panel of consultants. By March 25, he and Mary had garnered the senatorial support needed to plead their case to the Committee on Labor and Public Welfare.

"A medical dictionary defines cancer, which comes from the Latin word meaning crab, as 'a progressive growth of tissue,'" Yarborough began. "I prefer a more vivid definition of cancer given on the floor of the U.S. Senate more than 40 years ago by the late Senator Matt Neely . . . who died in 1958 of the very disease he had been fighting legislatively for more than three decades. . . . 'The name of this loathsome, deadly and insatiate monster is cancer.'"[23]

Yarborough noted that in the years since Neely had made that speech, three times as many Americans were now dying annually of the disease. He told the committee he planned to establish a panel of consultants on the conquest of cancer. The panel would have two primary tasks: first, to examine the adequacy and effectiveness of the present level of both governmental and nongovernmental support of cancer research, and second, to recommend to Congress and the American people what must be done to achieve cures for the major forms of cancer by 1976. The cost of the panel would not exceed $250,000, and their final report would be presented to the committee by January 31, 1971.

A concurrent resolution had been presented on the House side a few weeks earlier, and both were approved by a voice vote. Yarborough's phone call to Mary made it official. "Now, who will we appoint?" They had already agreed that the panel's composition had to be carefully crafted in order for their ultimate recommendations to be accepted and become law. Democrats held a majority; they would be no problem. Republican senator Javits was interested and could deliver the liberals of that party. But the conservatives were aligned with Nixon, so care would be needed to bring them on board. As Mary's original memo had suggested, the twenty-six-person panel would follow her familiar committee recipe: half lay members and half members from the medical-scientific world.

Waging the ultimate war against the "loathsome, deadly and insatiate monster," and then defeating it once and for all, was a thrilling prospect. But while everyone knew passing laws against the disease would *not* force it into submission, no one—not a member of Congress, not a representative from ACS or NCI, nor any of the crusade's medical allies—brought that up. Rather, the country's bicentennial year was set as *the* goal line for the cure of cancer. Period.

Chapter 12

~

"I'm Just a Catalytic Agent"

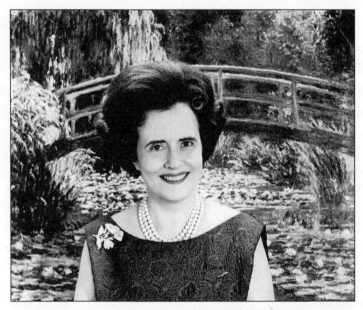

Mary in front of her favorite Monet painting,
The Japanese Footbridge and the Water Lily Pool, *circa 1960s.*

The letters were dated June 2, 1970. "As you know, the Senate has authorized this Committee [Labor and Public Welfare] to conduct a study of research activities in cancer. . . . I am authorized to appoint a Committee of Consultants. . . . I would personally appreciate it very much if you would agree to serve on this panel. . . . I hope you will accept this invitation . . . I am confident that your efforts will be well rewarded and that all mankind will benefit from them. Sincerely yours, Ralph W. Yarborough, Chairman."[1]

The recipients of these letters had been the product of numerous discussions between Mary and Yarborough. He had told her, "I only know one person I want, and that's Jubal Parten, a very nice businessman in Texas." Parten was indeed nice, and a successful and philanthropic Houston oilman who had donated to the senator's campaigns. The rest of the individuals on the panel were selected because of their bona fides in the cancer world and their respective businesses, along with their ability to deliver the wow factor in interviews to Congress or the media. Some were already well known; others would become giants. Mary knew them all, in person or by reputation.

The medical side included Sidney Farber, of course, and Dr. Lee Clark of M. D. Anderson. Yarborough liked that Clark was a fellow Texan who had also served on the DeBakey commission in 1965. Solomon Garb, whose book so inspired Mary, was selected, along with Dr. Joseph Burchenal, vice president of Memorial Sloan Kettering (MSK) in New York. He, in turn, recommended Dr. James Holland of Roswell Park Memorial Institute. Also from MSK was research assistant Dr. Mathilde Krim, whose husband, Arthur, was the former Democratic National Committee treasurer; both were good friends of Mary's. Dr. William Hutchinson, a pal of Senator Magnuson's and the founder of the Fred Hutchinson Cancer Research Center (named for his deceased, baseball-playing brother) was tapped, as was Dr. Paul Cornely, president of the American Public Health Association.

There was also a group from academia, including Dr. Jonathan Rhoads, a University of Pennsylvania faculty member and president of ACS, and Dr. Wendell Scott, from Washington University in St. Louis, who had been president of ACS and was now editor of its magazine. Selected from Stanford were geneticist Dr. Joshua Lederberg and radiologist Dr. Henry Kaplan, and, from the University of Wisconsin McCardle Laboratory for Cancer Research, Dr. Harold Rusch.

Besides Yarborough's choice of Parten, the lay members included other friends of Mary's: Foote, Anna Rosenberg Hoffman (she had remarried), Bill Blair, and Laurance Rockefeller, from whom Mary asked for assistance in selecting Republicans. He suggested Bobst (of course); G. Keith Funston, a former president of the New York Stock Exchange and another Nixon friend; and Benno Schmidt, a senior partner in the investment firm J. H. Whitney & Company and a member of the MSK board of trustees. It was important that the panel have members of both parties, so that it would be looked upon favorably by the Nixon administration. These were the days when political differences sometimes made for strange—and successful—bedfellows.

Rounding out the list were the industry people: Lew Wasserman, president of the Music Corporation of America (and a big Democratic contributor); Emil Mazey, the secretary-treasurer of the United Auto Workers; I. W. Abel, president of the United Steelworkers; Mary Wells Lawrence, chairperson of the advertising firm Wells, Rich, Greene; and Michael J. O'Neill, managing editor of the New York *Daily News*.

Having helped create the panel with Yarborough, Mary hadn't expected to receive an invitation letter addressed to her, nor the handwritten note at the bottom: "Dear Mary, Your letter should have been the *first* mailed. It was your genius, energy, and will to help mankind which created the committee. Please accept today. I think you should be our co-chairman, Ralph."[2]

The committee would be very much in the public eye, and that was certainly *not* Mary's style. Her participation, never mind the chairmanship, would have been, in her words, "a disaster." As she had long maintained, she wished always to remain in the background, never wanting credit for anything. She preferred to be the idea factory, pulling others in. "I'm just the catalytic agent," she insisted. And if the recommendations of the Committee of Consultants for the Conquest of Cancer (also referred to as the Panel of Consultants) led to a cure, it would surely be the biggest idea to ever come out of the "catalytic agent's" factory.

Not long after accepting his appointment to the panel, Rockefeller suggested to Mary that they consider Benno Schmidt for the chairmanship. It was because of Rockefeller that Schmidt was chairman of the board of trustees of MSK. Yarborough and Schmidt knew each other; although the latter had lived in the East for thirty years, he had been born in Abilene and attended the University of Texas and then Texas Law School. Yarborough had been one of his professors and was now very pleased at the suggestion to make his successful former student ("that fine young man from Abilene," as Yarborough called him) the panel's chair.[3] Before he accepted the position, Schmidt made inquiries. He wasn't afraid to take on bold new ventures, but he wanted to be certain this was a "serious" group. He found it was, and accepted, with Farber as co-chair.

Yarborough had lost the Texas primary election a month earlier. He had served fourteen years in the Senate and had loved doing so. Surely the loss must have given him moments of regret. But his defeat also meant the conquest of cancer could be his legacy, and now he could focus fully on it. Mary still needed more friends in the House, however. Her research about the full Appropriations Committee revealed that several of its members were part of the Democratic Study Group, a caucus of representatives created in 1959 that served as "a liberal counterpoint to the influence of senior conservatives and southern Democrats."[4] After a meeting with a number of the caucus members, and sharing her frustrations about medical research, Mary invited the entire group to another dinner party at the Blairs'. These social gatherings brought ample opportunities for an innocent mention of a current project, something she had learned long ago.

In the early fifties, she and Albert had hosted a pre-theater dinner party, inviting friends and her usual cabal of doctors. In their beautiful Beekman Place dining room, over a spread fit for royalty, Mary began a conversation about cancer research. Soon it dominated the room. Without missing a beat, Albert said, "All right, Mary, that's enough of that goddamn stuff about medical research. Let's just have a social evening."[5] He laughed, as did everyone else, and the dinner continued.

A decade later, Mary was still the ultimate connector. At the Blairs' dinner party, the Study Group members were joined by Farber, DeBakey, and other doctors who presented the current state of research, what had been accomplished, and what work still needed to be done. Once again, it was made clear that no one was beyond the terrifying grasp of the killer diseases. As it happened, one dinner guest, Representative James Corman, was very familiar with DeBakey's handiwork, having taken a good friend to him for open heart surgery. The dinner was a success, and Mary used it to forge new House alliances.

Luke Cornelius Quinn was a New Yorker. After serving in the Army Air Corps during World War II, he was assigned to the Air Force Legislative Liaison Office, a bureau whose work was to keep communication flowing on all subjects between those two bodies. In the course of his duties, he met fellow Irishman John Fogarty. A friendship developed between them. When Quinn retired from the military in 1951, Fogarty introduced him to Mary. Certainly someone with Quinn's extensive Capitol Hill experience and vast connections would be useful in their efforts, Fogarty suggested.[6] Mary agreed wholeheartedly; extra eyes and ears in Washington were always a good thing. She sent a check for $4,000 (about $44,000 today) to the New York office of the United Cerebral Palsy Association, one of the diseases her research lobby was championing at the time. The accompanying letter was to her friend Leonard Goldenson, co-founder of the association and president of United Paramount Theaters. In introducing Quinn, Mary suggested he take on a lobbying project, writing he was "to attempt to educate Congressmen and Senators . . . as to the needs of research." The money was for his salary, to be paid in "monthly installments."[7]

Quinn's initial work was impressive, and once he finished with the United Cerebral Palsy Association, Mary sent a check to her friend Lane Adams, executive vice president of ACS, with a similar accompanying letter. As time passed, people assumed that Quinn worked for ACS rather than the National Health Education Committee, of which Mary was chair. He was effective at coaching both legislators and witnesses, toting around copies of the current edition of the NHEC's Big Fact Book (this edition was titled *Does Medical Research Pay Off?*). Quinn used this book, filled with figures and charts, as his ultimate teaching tool. He fit into the crusade family perfectly.

In 1969, Quinn had begun to not feel well, and the news reached Mary. His abdominal symptoms sounded far too similar to Albert's early complaints, and Mary called Farber for advice. After a series of doctor visits, an exploratory surgery, and a diagnosis of gallbladder cancer, Quinn ended up at the NCI office of chemotherapy researcher, Dr. Vincent DeVita. After more tests, DeVita delivered the news that Quinn was, indeed, one of the more than 650,000 Americans who would be diagnosed with cancer that year. But the bright side was that Quinn did not have gallbladder cancer; rather, he had non-Hodgkin's lymphoma, which had been responding well to the new chemotherapy cocktail DeVita had been working on. Quinn began the difficult inpatient treatment at once. And from his NCI hospital room, he continued working on Mary's projects, one of which had been writing the text of the now famous "Dear Mr. Nixon" ad. At the end of his treatment, all signs of Quinn's lymphoma were gone. Mary was ecstatic, and not just because her friend had been given a new lease on life. Quinn had just become a living, breathing poster boy for her core beliefs that drugs could cure cancer.[8]

At the same time Quinn was finishing his chemotherapy regimen, Robert Sweek was listening to Dr. Garb on the radio. Garb was speaking about his book and making the defeat of cancer a national goal. Sweek was a program manager at the Atomic Energy Commission (AEC) and had just attended a conference on reframing large-scale technological programs for smaller, nongovernmental use. He wrote to Garb suggesting a similar application might be beneficial in cancer control. Additional friendly exchanges ensued, culminating in Sweek visiting Garb in Denver. The two men hit it off, and the doctor urged Sweek to meet Quinn in D.C. Quinn quickly understood Garb's enthusiasm for the man. A visit to Mary was next for Sweek, and on June 12, 1970, Yarborough announced Sweek's appointment as the staff director for the Panel of Consultants.[9] Since the goal was to create a program akin to the Manhattan Project (from which Sweek's employer, the AEC, had come) and an agency like NASA (in the creation of which Yarborough had played a part), it seemed a match made in heaven.

On June 29, the Panel of Consultants convened their inaugural meeting in Washington. A few members had asked that their participation only be titular; they wouldn't be attending meetings or voting. That was acceptable; their names on the report would still carry weight. The rest were ready to work, and Yarborough welcomed the group by reaffirming their deadline: cancer would be conquered by America's bicentennial. He asked the panel to aim for an October 31 report completion date, even though Congress had given them until the end of January 1971. During lunch, Schmidt and Farber outlined their thoughts on creating four subpanels: "Where do we stand?," "Where is good work going on and who is doing it?," "Delineation of areas of greatest promise," and "Mechanics for coordination, and promulgation of information." As panel members divided themselves up into the smaller groups, enthusiasm ran high, with three of the subpanels having initial meetings that same day.[10]

Mary was elated when she heard the panel had officially begun working. The ultimate impotence of the 1965 Heart Disease, Cancer, and Stroke Amendments had been disappointing. "It should have done what I'm talking about now," she said, "making the conquest of these diseases national goals. This commission for the conquest of cancer through research [is] going to be a second effort, a big effort!"

The week prior, Mary had received a letter from her friend Lister Hill. After bringing her up to date on an event he had attended, he told her, "I want to say again that you stand at the forefront of Florence Nightingale, [Red Cross founder] Clara Barton, Madame Curie and Helen Taussig [founder of pediatric cardiology] in your wonderful contributions to the health of our people and to the health of all mankind."[11] His kindness meant a great deal to her. As those women had, she lived in a world completely dominated by men. Misogyny still echoed through the halls of Congress, where only eleven women were among the 535 total members. Just 8 percent of the previous decade's medical school graduates were women, and only 6.7 percent of all practicing physicians were female. Women in science made up a paltry 19 percent across all disciplines.[12]

Mary had never looked through a microscope, performed surgery, or spoken from the floor of the Capitol. She simply had an unbridled belief in possibility. That undying confidence aside, however, this would be her toughest battle yet.

For President Nixon, the first half of 1970 was one bad month after another. Vietnam was a maddening nightmare; roughly 335,000 U.S. troops were still in-country.[13] His policy of "Vietnamization"—meant to "expand, equip, and train South Vietnamese forces" so that U.S. combat troops could be drawn down— was not working as successfully as he had hoped. In a perverted dichotomy, a Valentine's Day Gallup poll showed that 55 percent of Americans opposed an immediate withdrawal from South Vietnam, yet the anti-war demonstrations grew in size and frequency, culminating in the horrific May deaths of four students on Ohio's Kent State University campus.[14] These home front challenges suggested that perhaps domestic policy was not as simple as the president had originally thought. In addition to ongoing fears of leaks from within the administration and other government agencies, Nixon had become bothered by Secretary Finch's hesitancy to accept the health budgets he submitted. In June, Finch resigned, stepping into the role of counselor to the president. Elliot Richardson became the new department secretary.

Mike Gorman liked Richardson, reporting to Mary that he seemed to be interested in mental health problems. That was at least something. Although she found Richardson energetic, Mary also thought he was rather cold, and remarked he'd probably manage the department along Republican lines. There had also been an equally important change at NCI. After nine years, Kenneth Endicott had stepped down as agency head. Dr. Carl Baker was made acting director, and after an extensive search, his appointment was made permanent. Endicott had not been a fan of applied research. Baker was, however, and particularly intent on solving the problem of cancer. He did not, though, have experience dealing with Congress. Regardless of Mary's thoughts and feelings about these men, they would be the ones at the forefront when the Panel of Consultants made their report.

The group's second meeting was on July 27, during which the subpanels gave updates on their work. Then, on his way to the third meeting, on August 24, Farber suffered a mild coronary. He had had a similar event five years earlier, but this time he heeded his body's signals and, after forty-one years, stepped down as a Harvard faculty member. He would also need to take a leave from his responsibilities as co-chair of the panel (although he would be back by the time they made their presentation). With the full panel's agreement, Schmidt asked Dr. Clark to step in for Farber.

Much of the panel's final report would be technical and would draw on the expertise of the scientific members. Schmidt realized a full-time coordinator would be needed to pull it all together, and he asked panel member and MSK oncologist Dr. Burchenal to step into that role. Schmidt also decided to get an advance read on the thoughts of members of Congress regarding the panel's work. He scheduled meetings with some, and then asked House minority leader Gerald Ford, a Republican, to organize a luncheon for September 16. Schmidt and Burchenal joined seven congressmen representing both political parties. Following the luncheon, Schmidt also met with George Shultz, who was the director of the Office of Management and Budget and, more importantly, a presidential advisor on domestic policy. It was all a brilliant way to set the stage.

The suggestion that a new organization might be required to conquer cancer had first come up in Yarborough's March speech on the Senate floor, when he proposed the formation of the panel "with particular attention directed toward the creation of a new administrative agency."[15] After multiple conversations between Schmidt, Sweek, Quinn, and Burchenal, that subject became the main topic at the September panel meeting. It was a radical idea, and there were dissenters among the group. They had agreed at the outset that their final recommendations had to be unanimous. This issue had to be resolved quickly; the clock was ticking toward the October 31 deadline for the completion of their report. Sweek was concerned, but Quinn told him not to worry; the no votes would change.[16] As had been the case in the famed 1957 Sidney Lumet movie *12 Angry Men*, educated persuasion would be necessary, and that was Quinn's specialty.

Logically put, if their ultimate goal of the eradication of cancer was not being achieved via the existing agency structure, they *must* consider options. They *must* take on NIH. Schmidt drew up a draft recommending the creation of a new body to serve as a national cancer authority, and circulated it among the panel members. After myriad meetings, memos, and phone calls, by the time the group reconvened on October 7, they were 100 percent in agreement about the new entity.

Although the media hadn't paid much attention to the panel's creation in the spring of 1970, by mid-July a weekly health and medicine newsletter had created a firestorm. *The Blue Sheet* (a publication of *Drug Research Reports*) wasn't shy about colorfully describing the meetings as "closed-door" and "secret hearings." "Battle lines between 'creative research' and 'structured research'" were being drawn, the author wrote, and the whole thing was being "modeled after the applied and developmental systems approach used by AEC and NASA." As the weeks went by, more *Blue Sheet* articles stirred the pot.[17] In August and November, the *Wall Street Journal* wrote about the panel, too, albeit with less incendiary words: "The committee . . . may at least answer that question that many Americans asked a year ago when Neil Armstrong stepped on the moon: 'If we can land men on the moon, why can't we find a cure for cancer?'"[18]

Sandwiched in between the *Wall Street Journal* pieces, an October *Science* magazine article bore the headline "Cancer Research: Senate Consultants Likely to Push for Planned Assault." The author doubted that "a program calling for massive spending on cancer research will have presidential support." But he also noted that "the Yarborough commission recommendations may . . . affect the manner in which the current level of funding for cancer is administered."[19]

This made the scientific community prick up its ears. It wasn't against the concept of cancer research. But money was a different story. Who would get it, and who would decide how it would be spent? Mary had long declared that too many levels existed in the NIH funding process. When scientists wanted to pursue an idea, committees and offices held discussions about it. Since the requested funds came from the federal government, PHS, HEW, Congress, the Office of Management and Budget, and ultimately the president himself were involved, using up valuable time for both patients and the scientists. New NCI director Baker found even the hiring process the ultimate in frustration. It, too, was layered like a mille-feuille pastry. By the time qualified candidates were finally approved, they had often given up waiting and moved on to positions elsewhere. But Baker was not in favor of unlinking NCI and NIH.[20]

Mary had remained in the background throughout the panel's work. First Farber and then Foote served as her proxy. Foote let Sweek know in mid-October that Mary wanted to see the report, even if it wasn't completely polished.

Schmidt and Rockefeller brought it to her personally, prior to the panel's final meeting on October 30. She found two issues that needed immediate correction. First, she wanted the proposed National Cancer Advisory Board (similar to what currently existed at NCI) to have the final word of approval on all research contracts. That had been a problem when Endicott was director. A compromise was struck: the board would oversee contracts the first year, and the new agency's administrator would take on that task moving forward.

The second issue, however, brooked no compromise; it was completely non-negotiable. Mary wanted specific verbiage that spoke to a substantial and rapid increase in funds for cancer research and included the actual budget numbers. She had learned the lesson that using vague language to refer to amounts ensured disappointment. The Panel of Consultants was completely on board with this request. Without specific funds solidly in place, this legislation would be no different from any other rhetoric on cancer that had come out of Washington over the years.

Meanwhile, the public guessing game of what might come from the panel continued. "A massive infusion of money" was what seemed to be most expected. Asked about Yarborough's promise to eliminate cancer by 1976, Sweek told the writer what he had heard from the panel's medical members: "If we had a cure today, we couldn't prove it out by 1976." Their goal, nonetheless, was to at least have a cure in hand. Another article pointed out that the cancer problem was complicated by the fact there were "more than 100" varieties of the disease. Furthermore, scientists still didn't understand what made cells go rogue in the first place. The article finished with one of Mary's favorite mantras: "If the assault isn't stepped up now, the conquest of the disease will only be delayed that much longer."[21]

⟶

"I began talking my White House diary into a tape recorder two or three days after November 22, 1963," Lady Bird Johnson wrote in the prologue of her newly published book, *White House Diary*.[22] Debuting in early November 1970 at a whopping 806 pages, the book was all anyone who was anyone could talk about. LBJ intercepted the first copy that arrived at their Texas ranch. The Johnsons had invited Mary and Laurance and Mary Rockefeller for the weekend. At dinner that first night, the former president produced the book with much flourish and toasted his wife with pride.[23] Then at the end of the month, Mary held a party of her own for Lady Bird at Beekman Place. An autograph session was combined with a bon voyage soirée before the former First Lady took her book tour to London.

Twelve days later (on Friday, December 4, 1970), meteorologists told Washington residents to expect a few rain showers. Had they known what was about to be presented to the Senate Committee on Labor and Public Welfare, they might have upped their prediction to a full-blown hurricane. That morning, Senator Yarborough made his way from his office in the Old Senate Office Building (which would be renamed the following year to honor Georgia's senator Richard Russell Jr.) to the Dirksen Senate Office Building. His footsteps echoed in the building's marble foyer but were muted when he reached the plush carpet of the ornately paneled hearing room. The committee members sat at a long table at the front of the room, with a speaker's lectern facing them. Behind the lectern was a small coterie that included Schmidt, Farber, Clark, and Mary.

Once they were called to order, Senator Yarborough addressed his fellow members. "I introduce for appropriate reference a bill which would establish a National Cancer Authority. . . . During my years in public service I always have been guided by the principle so eloquently stated by Thomas Jefferson, 'The care of human life and happiness and not their destruction, is the first and only legitimate object of good government.'"[24]

While no one would have argued the horror of cancer, Yarborough read through figures relating to the disease anyway, all of which came from Mary. In fact, the majority of the panel's report had been written by Quinn and overseen by Mary. The senator next introduced the panel members, praising them for their work, and then spoke directly to Jacob Javits—the ranking member of the full Committee on Labor and Public Welfare—calling him a "partner" in this project and expressing hope that Javits would carry on after Yarborough's departure. The Republican from New York confirmed with gusto that he would.

Committee member Ted Kennedy suggested that his fellow members bear in mind the vote that had taken place the previous day regarding government funding of the Super Sonic Transport (SST). President Nixon and his administration had been big supporters of this program. But the Senate voted to discontinue its funding, giving many, including Kennedy, a reason to celebrate. Noise and exhaust pollution had been cited as SST's negatives; however, an additional theme in the congressional debate had also included suggestions that funding intended for an "expensive technological project of dubious value" be reallocated for pressing domestic issues.[25] Cancer certainly fell into the latter category. With these seemingly innocent remarks, Kennedy fired the first salvo that put cancer in the middle of what would become a political war.

Schmidt came to the podium and began to read the panel's recommendations. "First. Establish an independent agency to be known as the National Cancer Authority. This agency would be directed by an Administrator and Deputy Administrator, appointed by the president, with the advice and consent of the Senate, for terms of 5 years."[26]

This radical idea carried many messages. It said the panel had no confidence in NIH. It said that the organization's bureaucracy curtailed the efficiency of cancer research. It said cancer had not been given the priority due it, considering the millions who died of the disease each year and the greater number diagnosed. And it said a new and independent agency would escape the agonizing budget cuts routinely made by NIH and HEW. Mary hoped those messages would echo often in the coming months.

"Second. Transfer to the National Cancer Authority all of the functions of the National Cancer Institute."[27] Everything within and being done by NCI would now fall under the purview of the new agency and its new National Cancer Advisory Council (the words in the NACC's name were frequently rearranged to the National Cancer Advisory Council, but it was the same body with the same mission). This section also gave the NCAC a voice in contracts and grants. Another shock.

"Third. Charge the National Cancer Authority with the responsibilities of conducting research and utilizing existing research facilities in the search for a cure for cancer."[28] Less shocking, but still radical.

"Fourth. Establish a National Cancer Advisory Board of 18 members, nine scientists or physicians, and nine representatives of the general public appointed by the president, with the advice and consent of the Senate. . . . We authorize $400 million to begin research in this area immediately, with increases of up to $1 billion a year as soon as possible."[29] This was probably the least radical recommendation, but the amount suggested was staggering.

Kennedy praised the panel's work as "an example of the cooperation that was possible between public and private health sectors." He asked Schmidt if, considering his extensive business acumen, the panel chair thought the country could afford the program they had suggested. "My strong personal view," Schmidt responded, "is not only can we afford this effort, we cannot afford not to do it."[30]

Bills based on the panel's recommendations were introduced in both the Senate and the House. But coming so near the end of the congressional session, and with other pressing items on the docket, the Conquest of Cancer Act (officially known as S. 4564) would not be further discussed until January. By that time, Yarborough would be gone. His replacement as chair of the Labor and Public Welfare committee hadn't yet been decided. But Kennedy promised to take up the charge, nonetheless.

On December 8, NIH director Marston issued a memo to HEW assistant secretary Egeberg. "I have responded, after talking with you, to reporters asking my views on the subject report, prepared by the National Panel of Consultants on the Conquest of Cancer," Marston wrote, noting that the panelists "have given unselfishly of their time and talents" and that he concurred "in their recommendation of enhanced support of research." He also recognized that their "proposed enhanced financing" would not be "at the expense of other research programs."

However, he added, "the unequivocal disagreement I have is the proposed locus of cancer research activity in a separate agency." Marston went on to explain that much of the panel's impetus for creating the new organization was already available within NCI. And if they needed something else, they could simply go to Congress and request it. He pointed out that various institutes and divisions were already working on the "areas of specific promise listed by the Panel." He specifically referred to virologists, immunologists, cell biologists, epidemiologists, pharmacologists, and others focusing on "fundamental life processes." That was a reference to basic research, not Mary's favorite. "The NIH," she later described indignantly, "has been philosophically, totally opposed to bringing any scientific answers to people. They just want to be a storehouse of information and basic research. They decided it wasn't their mission."

Marston went on to say that while there had been a "leveling off of research dollars since 1967," too much money would "overload facilities and tax expert manpower. . . . The expansion of research support should be phased up on the basis of manpower available." This appeared to be another chicken-or-egg problem. There wasn't enough money for more researchers or larger facilities, but making more money available would be futile if they didn't have the researchers or facilities.

He finished with, "The NIH will explore responsively the several recommendations of the report regarding improved coordination and integration . . . that should be sought in order to pursue research objectives in cancer." Marston seemed surprised that there were coordination problems. If there were, surely NCI director Baker would have previously shared his frustrations at wading through the bureaucracy to hire new talent.[31]

Over the days after Yarborough's original presentation, an identical Associated Press distillation of the recommendations ran in papers across the country. A December 14 editorial in the *Charlotte Observer* viewed the act favorably, pointing out the previous year's federal expenditures (supplied by Mary, of course): "For every man, woman and child in America, the United States last year saw $410 for general defense, $125 for Vietnam in particular, and about $20 for the space program. The per capita spending for cancer research was only $0.89."[32]

Those startling comparisons drove home the point for more research. But Mary was focused on journalist Judith Randal's article in the December 12

Washington Star. Randal called the idea of an agency separate from NIH "questionable" and complex. She didn't feel that the comparison of the National Cancer Authority to the Manhattan Project or NASA had been thoroughly thought through. Equally important, Randal felt that creating the authority would exacerbate warfare among health causes: "If cancer—which already gets top-priority funding at the expense of such relatively neglected disorders as arthritis—became even more privileged, the bitterness would intensify."[33]

These would be but two of the winds that would blow against the panel's recommendations. Ever the optimist, Mary brushed them aside, saying of Randal's points, "I think her questions can easily be answered, and I'm hoping that we'll get this legislation by early summer." After all, as Farber had pointed out the previous year, not long ago physicians had thought that cancer was just an "incontestable feature of nature." Yet here they were, expressing "restrained optimism" that the question of cancer could be solvable.

Mary had thought often about the NASA comparison. In 1964, she had told an interviewer, "It's not that I think that less should be done to explore space. It's just that space research costs so much more in proportion to the total economy." Now, six years later, she calculated all that would be needed to rid the world of cancer was a small fraction of the $24 billion it had cost taxpayers for the trip to the moon. The "few pounds of rocks and soil of interest to a handful of physical scientists"—as a *Wall Street Journal* writer described the items brought back as a result of the Apollo 11 landing—did not impact the nation's bottom line.[34] But according to Mary's then-current version of "Does Research Pay Off?" "The median age at death has increased from 63.4 in 1943 to 70.6. These added years of life, as well as the reduction in the disabilities achieved through medical research advances, are certainly a major factor in the increase in our gross national product."

There was another interesting thread connecting the Manhattan Project, NASA, and cancer, one that had not yet been addressed in print: fear. After World War II, the threat of Nazism had given way to the threat of Communism. The Manhattan Project had become the AEC, which would continue to experiment with the powerful weaponry for more than two decades. The Soviets, too, had been experimenting, and successfully tested an atomic bomb in August 1949. Overnight, nuclear world annihilation became a real possibility.

The Soviets began working on space travel, too, launching the world's first satellite in 1957. America would answer in January 1958. The Soviets were also the first to send a human into space in April 1961 (twenty-three days before NASA's first Mercury launch). Again, fear spawned questions about the Soviets' intentions. Yet cancer was still listed as the nation's greatest fear. While Americans wanted to stop the spread of Communism, in a 1969 survey they listed cancer as being a problem more vital than world poverty or the Vietnam War. In light of that, why *not* a cancer moon shot?

Chapter 13

"We Can All Share in the Eventual Glory"

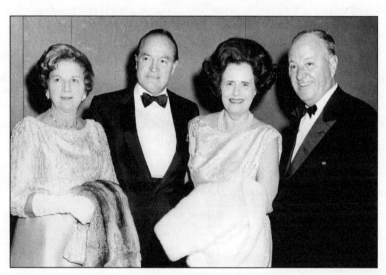

Mary at the American College of Physicians Humanitarian Award dinner with Bob Hope and Mr. and Mrs. Joseph Martino, 1965.

The house at 29 Beekman Place was even more beautiful than usual on Saturday, December 6, 1970. It was a festive blaze of light for Mary's annual Christmas party. Every room was festooned with live greenery, white lilies, and white roses. Mantels were decked with garlands, and Christmas trees abounded. And "the catalytic agent" maintained her practice of entertaining with a purpose: celebrities and socialites mingled with doctors and crusade members.

Mary's longtime friend Eleanor Lambert was in attendance and was eloquent in her description of the hostess in her next column. "Thinking back over the good things that have happened during the tumultuous past ten years," she wrote, "no one could fail to be amazed at how many of them grew out of the planning and prodding . . . and friendly but persistent persuasion that is Mary Lasker's subtle art."[1]

That "art" had translated into NIH's astounding budget growth over the decade: from $560 million in fiscal 1961 to $1.8 billion in fiscal 1971. Eleanor had also witnessed Mary's clever use of the power of the public. Without a White House ally, she explained, "Mrs. Lasker is at present working with her usual low-keyed dedication to inspire a mammoth public appeal to President Nixon to make the conquest of cancer a national goal."

She gave Mary's crusade a plug, quoting her directly: "If people everywhere would take a moment to write to the president and remind him that the smallest fraction of the cost of putting another team on the moon may mean the end of both cancer and heart disease as the greatest killers of humanity, we can all share in the eventual glory."

The glory, Mary hoped, would be achieved in the next decade. What would those ten years hold? According to ACS, the future looked grim: 6.5 million new cases of cancer would be diagnosed in those ten years, 3.5 million people would die of the disease, and more than 10 million people would be in some stage of treatment.[2] Oblivious to these predictions, and for the second year in a row, Nixon's budget proposal had cut funding for cancer research from the requested $300 million to $180 million. The budget cuts would be further impacted by the federal shift in focus from research to increase numbers of medical personnel.

Organizational changes, too, were in the works. Over the past few years, NIH had inherited responsibility for the Bureau of Health Manpower, the National Library of Medicine, and the National Eye Institute. Meanwhile, the massive National Institute of Mental Health and the Regional Medical Program had been moved out, taking their budgets with them. This caused NIH (and by extension NCI) to have to compete even more rigorously for dollars.

How wonderful it would be if Americans could enter the 1980s without the specter of cancer hanging over their heads. Could the Panel of Consultants' goal of a cure for cancer by 1976 be met?

⌐

Weeks earlier, when Ted Kennedy had cast a vote against continuing the SST funding and then suggested reallocation of the dollars, President Nixon took notice. He was a big proponent of the SST. And he took assaults on his policies personally, determining that *his* next targeted assault would carry the same sting. He didn't have to wait long. On December 16, both chambers of Congress had overwhelmingly passed the Family Practice of Medicine Act to rectify the short-age of family practitioners, particularly in rural areas of the country. Senator Yarborough had been strongly in favor of it, and Kennedy had co-sponsored the bill. Nixon, therefore, conceived of a clever and controversial way to squelch it.

After a bill passes in both chambers of Congress, it's sent to the Oval Office. The president has ten days to sign it or veto it; the president can also do nothing, in which case the bill becomes law. However, if Congress is not in session at the end of that ten-day period, there would be no one for the president to return the bill to, and it would die, having been "pocket-vetoed." That was the option Nixon chose, as Congress had departed for its holiday recess. Kennedy was incensed, so much so that he filed a lawsuit against the administration. Even though the suit would not be heard for two years, Kennedy never took lightly an attack against health care for Americans.[3]

What drove Kennedy's interest in health care is hard to pinpoint. He al-luded to his mother's emphasis on health and her meticulous record-keeping of her children's illnesses and doctor visits. The senator was also moved by a sister's mental health challenges, Jack's physical challenges, and his father's 1961 stroke. But his own severe injuries in a June 1964 plane crash really whetted his appetite for the subject. His long convalescence in hospitals, surrounded by medical professionals, gave him ample time to learn from them and study the nation's health care issues more closely. As had been true for Mary years earlier, Kennedy realized that illness and injury care did not come cheap. The lack of funds to cover medical costs was a devastating reality to middle- and lower-income Americans.[4]

Kennedy had become the Democratic majority whip in 1969 (the youngest senator to achieve the position) but lost it in January 1971 to Robert Byrd of West Virginia. Meanwhile, when Yarborough left the Senate—and the chairmanship of both the Labor and Public Welfare Committee and its Subcommittee on Health and Scientific Research—Mary worried about the vacancies. She had hoped that Senator Harrison Williams of New Jersey would be made chairman of the entire committee, and he was. Her second wish was for Kennedy to take on the chair of the subcommittee. "If Teddy's the chairman it will be wonderful," she said at the time. "He really has a feel for health."

Mary's second wish was granted, too. Kennedy would later tell Byrd that the majority whip defeat was a blessing to him, as he felt his strengths lay in committee work, where he could pursue his personal interests.[5] It was a blessing to the crusade as well. Mary had a long history with the Kennedy family. But there was a special place in her heart for Ted.

As the first session of the Ninety-second Congress was set to begin on January 21, Quinn informed Mary that Kennedy, along with Republican senator Jacob Javits, was ready to introduce S. 34 on the twenty-sixth. It was the same bill Yarborough had introduced in December, based on the panel's recommendations, but renumbered to reflect the new congressional calendar. The culmination of decades of work was finally going to see daylight. But dark clouds were just over the horizon. And riding on those clouds was political intrigue the likes of which had never before been seen in the realm of the nation's health.

⁓

"Reds Attack Cambodian Capital."

"Richard Russell, Dean of All Senators, Dies at 73."

"Democrats Oust Kennedy as Whip."

Of these attention-grabbing headlines on January 22, one gave Richard Nixon greater pleasure than the grief of the other two combined. If Kennedy's own party hadn't supported him as majority whip, maybe they wouldn't support him as a presidential candidate, either. The prospect of running against another Kennedy gnawed at Nixon day and night.[6] But that worry was a waste of the president's time, as Ted Kennedy absolutely did *not* want the presidency in 1972. He had watched his brothers die because of the position. He had taken on the responsibility for their combined thirteen children, in addition to his own three. And he enjoyed his work in the Senate. Yet Nixon saw that every time the media fueled the fire of interest in Ted as a candidate, Kennedy rose higher in the polls.

On this particular morning, the president was putting the finishing touches on his second State of the Union address, the nation's 187th, which he would deliver that night at nine o'clock. As had now become common, the address, presented to the full Congress, would be televised. Back in December, Elmer Bobst—at the urging of Mary and Benno Schmidt—had used the occasion of his annual White House birthday party to suggest that Nixon mention the cancer initiative in his message.

Nixon was well aware of the cancer bill, which Kennedy planned to introduce in four days. His speech's focus would be on domestic problems and would be, as Nixon had told the press, "by far the most comprehensive, the most far-reaching, the most bold program in the domestic field ever presented to an American Congress."[7] Why not get ahead of the game? Why not grab cancer out from under the senator's nose?

"Mr. Speaker," Nixon began his message that night, "before I begin my formal address, I want to use this opportunity to congratulate all of those who were winners in the rather spirited contest for leadership positions in the House and the Senate and, also, to express my condolences to the losers. I know how both of you feel."[8] It was the perfect blend of attempted humor and a jab at Kennedy's loss of the majority whip post.

Mary was watching the address from her Palm Springs winter retreat as Nixon outlined his six goals for the "New American Revolution." He was a third of the way through when an announcement shocked her.

"I will also ask for an appropriation of an extra $100 million to launch an intensive campaign to find a cure for cancer, and I will ask later for whatever additional funds can effectively be used. The time has come in America when the same kind of concentrated effort that split the atom and took man to the moon should be turned toward conquering this dread disease. Let us make a total national commitment to achieve this goal."[9]

His use of the four phrases "cure for cancer," "split the atom," "took man to the moon," and "national commitment" should have been gratifying to Mary. They came straight out of the panel's report. But the president ignored the rest of their recommendations. And who was he kidding, offering up $100 million more? Certainly not Mary. Nixon's budget office (at his direction) had already cut $120 million off the requested $300 million for cancer research in that fiscal year. His promise of an additional $100 million brought the total proposed allocation for cancer research up to $280 million—$20 million short of the original amount asked for. It was a sham. Americans not involved in the crusade would never be aware that he was playing a deadly game, offering artificial benevolence for political gain.

The karma gods were paying attention, however. The newspaper stories the next day spoke of Nixon's cancer plan, calling it his "war on cancer." They also included the fact that Senator Edward Kennedy would be introducing a bill with the very same mission, a national "conquer cancer drive."[10] And in explaining the drive, the stories summed up the recommendations of the Panel of Consultants—recommendations presented *to* President Nixon, not suggested *by* him.

On January 26, as he had promised, Kennedy presented to the Senate the Conquest of Cancer Act. Hearings on the bill would begin in early March. Now, newspapers proclaimed that Ted Kennedy had just declared war on cancer, too. Despite the fact that neither man had said it, the phrase "war on cancer" stuck.[11] The same day he introduced S. 34, Kennedy also introduced S. 3, the Health Security Act, a $41 billion initiative calling for cradle-to-grave national health insurance. Nixon was livid and summoned John Ehrlichman, his domestic affairs advisor. A longtime friend of Nixon's who had worked on all of his campaigns, Ehrlichman listened to Nixon's plan to co-opt the senator's health initiatives. The president instructed his advisor to "hold back the Kennedy plan" and to pave the way for his administration to "get credit for what he [Kennedy] proposed and what passed."[12]

"He's a prisoner of the AMA, which raised a million and a half dollars for him through one of their non-tax-deductible funds." Mary had more assumptions than just this one regarding why she was expecting Nixon not to support S. 34. The AMA had long ago joined with the Republicans to prevent the government from involvement in medicine. "And since sixty percent of all surgery is cancer related," she asked angrily, "what would happen if you could really control cancer with drugs or vaccines or some other therapy?" Then, she sarcastically answered her own question: "That would be terrible for members of the AMA who are surgeons."

But there were other forces ramping up to work against the Conquest of Cancer Act. First, as Mary reported, "six members of the president's staff are Christian Scientists, and they are totally opposed to medicine and research in medicine." The six she mentioned included Ehrlichman and Bob Haldeman, Nixon's chief of staff, who ironically would die of colon cancer in 1993 at the age of sixty-seven, after refusing medical treatment.

The bigger battle would be waged by the science world, which had only just begun to "freak out"—to use a phrase gaining in popularity at the time. Their primary concern was the bill's (and the Panel of Consultants') very first recommendation: that to be most effective in the conquest of cancer, NCI would be renamed the National Cancer Authority and taken out of NIH. While direct quotes from NIH staff members were at a minimum in late January, Robert Marston told one journalist, "Cancer research profits from interplay with other research in the diseases of man."[13] That simple objection was only the breeze before the real storm.

And then, of course, there were the senators themselves. Their approval would be needed to move the bill forward, followed by House of Representatives approval. Anyone's opposition to an investment in the nation's health confounded Mary. "They think money is more important than life, or than preventing illness," she announced with exasperation. "There are some people who don't believe in research or that there will be any results from the money invested. They have had no experience with illness themselves or with anybody they cared about. Maybe they don't care about anybody. These are the things I don't understand!"

Mary had always been able to look beyond what her eyes alone could see. Now she could tell that there was a massive war brewing. And she was not about to fall behind the curve on this, the most passionate mission on which she'd ever embarked. Mary wanted all one hundred senators to be very clear about S. 34's benefit to humanity, so in the last week of January, she rallied Anna Hoffman and Laurance Rockefeller to accompany her to the office of Democratic senator Mike Mansfield of Montana. The three asked if he would give a Senate luncheon, which Mary would pay for, and during which the proposals in the bill could be explained prior to the bill coming up for official discussion. They wanted to be sure that the Senate was enthusiastic about it, and would pass it overwhelmingly. Mansfield was typically willing to work with his Republican counterparts, and said he'd host the lunch if they could persuade his Republican colleague from Pennsylvania, Hugh Scott, to co-host, explaining, "I don't want to make it seem like a partisan matter." Rockefeller went immediately to the office of Senator Scott, who readily agreed to co-host. They set the date for Thursday, February 11.

During the lunch, key members of the Panel of Consultants made statements, all choreographed from an agenda. Joining Schmidt were Drs. Farber, Clark, and Holland, plus Anna. After the doctors' remarks, Anna spoke from a human point of view, not about the science but about the suffering cancer caused. She made an effective and lasting impression.

Mary calculated that around three dozen senators attended the lunch. There would have been more, but it was the day before Lincoln's Birthday, and many had gone home to make speeches. Nonetheless, questions were asked of the panel members, and she could feel the enthusiasm running through the room.

Kennedy and Humphrey approached her afterward. "Listen," they told her, "this is going to take a lot of publicity and a lot of doing." Mary later said, "They had the feeling that there was going to be resistance to spending large amounts of money. And I figured, if they felt this way, being as astute as they are, they were surely right. So I told them I'd get them on the air." She had expected that the new National Cancer Authority was going to be the biggest issue of S. 34. If they could get public support for the funds early on, they'd have one less fight on their hands.

Getting the airtime would be easy for Mary. However, both senators' press staffs said no to the invitation, mumbling something about scheduling. Mary wasn't buying that, since the senators themselves were keen to go on the air. She surmised that the press staffs were envious of her media connections. Other offers of staff members who could speak for the senators were made available; however, the radio and TV stations only wanted the real thing.

Luke Quinn went to work immediately after the luncheon. His task was to visit both the senators who'd been there and, more importantly, those who hadn't, to garner additional co-sponsors and support for S. 34. That would help, but Mary was still nervous. Mary greatly admired the political acuity of Kennedy and Humphrey. The fact that they were concerned about opposition weighed heavily on her. It was so much on her mind that it followed her to one of her favorite annual rituals: every February, Mary (coming usually from Palm Springs) and her sister (coming from New York) met in the middle, at the luxurious Greenhouse Spa, run by Neiman Marcus's Stanley Marcus, just outside of Dallas.

During their stay at the spa, Mary shared with Alice her concerns about getting the word out about the benefits of the cancer bill. Alice told her that Ann Landers (whose real name was Eppie Lederer) had just written a column about the importance of breast self-exams. That had generated 250,000 requests to ACS for copies of the instructional pamphlet mentioned in the column. Alice suggested that perhaps Mary, who knew Lederer, could ask her to do something similar regarding the cancer bill. It was a brilliant idea. Mary would get the ball rolling as soon as she was back in New York.

Conquering cancer had probably been the least important thing on President Nixon's agenda on January 1. Now, on February 1, aside from keeping Ted

Kennedy off the ballot in 1972, cancer had become the most important thing to him. It was a bizarre version of a scene between archrival department store icons R. H. Macy and Bernard Gimbel in the holiday classic *Miracle on 34th Street*.

In that scene, Gimbel (who would be Nixon) says, "Every shopper in New York now thinks of Macy [who would be Kennedy] as a benevolent soul, thinking of nothing but the welfare of the public. And what does that make Gimbel? Nothing but a profiteering money-grubber. Well, two can play at that game." A joint photo op follows shortly afterward, whereupon Macy gives Santa a check (this would be the Conquest of Cancer bill). Gimbel asks what Santa will do with it. Santa replies that he'd like to give it to a doctor who needs a new X-ray machine. Macy says the check won't cover it, and offers to up the amount.

Gimbel jumps in to say, "I'll make up the difference."

Macy counters, "Buy it through the store and get a 10 percent discount."

Gimbel retorts, "I can get it for cost."

The comparison would be humorous were it not for the fact that the scene unfolding in Washington, D.C., was a matter of life and death. Nixon had announced "a total national commitment" to curing cancer, after which Kennedy introduced a bill to do the same thing. On February 18, the president upped the ante with a murky plan delivered in his annual health strategy message to Congress. He proposed that a Cancer Conquest Program be established at NIH, with the program's lead reporting to NIH director Marston. Marston was quoted in a subsequent newspaper article as saying that he would then convey relevant program information "concerning both plans and progress of the whole broad area of the cancer effort" to HEW and the president. Furthermore, Marston explained, the new program would be small and administrative, rather than operational.[14]

Marston made one final point very clear in his summation of the president's announcement: the new program would remain at NIH "in recognition that cancer research involves more of our institutes than just the National Cancer Institute." This appeared to leave even NCI director Baker confused: "As near as I can tell, the purpose [of the president's plan] is how to coordinate across institute lines, which I thought we were already doing. I don't know a lot more about it than that."

It was hardly what the Panel of Consultants and S. 34 had called for to conquer one of Americans' greatest fears and the second-greatest killer, as Kennedy quickly pointed out. "The administration's cancer initiative is a pale imitation of what we really need to conquer cancer," Kennedy said. "We cannot succeed simply by retaining the National Institutes of Health status quo."[15]

Dr. Vincent DeVita, then the chief of NCI's medical branch, saw through the charade, too. "There was never any coordination of research effort among the institutes at that time," he later said, "and very little research relevant to cancer was carried on outside the NCI."[16] Yet over the next ten months, this straw man would become the opposition's most frequent target, just as Mary had suspected.

The president had deliberately been vague, leaving elaboration to his science advisor, Dr. Edward E. David Jr. David was resolutely opposed to a new agency. He did not believe in an AEC- or NASA-type organization for cancer, and told an audience at a meeting of the Association of American Medical Colleges (AAMC) that Nixon felt the same. "It is the president's belief that having honed and sharpened our biomedical research mechanism, the National Institutes of Health, we should now use it."

He spoke of all the glorious achievements of NIH: "Vaccines for poliomyelitis, German measles, mumps and other infections are available to us all. . . . Children who would have been dead from leukemia are alive today and are regarded as cured in a surprising number of instances." Successes in overcoming Parkinson's disease, tuberculosis, and malaria were all the product of NIH. In listing these medical marvels, what he failed to mention was that the institutes that had developed them, and the funds that paid for their research, were often the result of Mary Lasker's work. Yet he did make an oblique reference to her, saying that while laypeople were not qualified to direct the research, the public was entitled "to know the strategy and the short-term objectives, and to receive progress reports."

David was also adamant regarding the notion that cancer could be tamed by the time the nation's bicentennial arrived—an idea that many (including, to his chagrin, the president) were espousing. "Cancer is not a simple disease; it is probably many," he said. "There is likely not to be a single cure, but a series of steps."[17] Wasn't that the very point of ramping up the research? Mary was confounded by the reticence of these people who were supposed to be dedicated to finding answers. "Since nobody knows the full picture of cancer," she asked, "how does anyone know what's an unrealistic demand and what isn't?" In other words, why was the administration dragging its feet?

Perhaps it was because the president was becoming ever more paranoid. In addition to a hostile Congress, Nixon felt even those within his administration might be against him. To address his fears, two days before giving his health message he had installed a taping system in the Oval Office, with five microphones concealed in his desk, two more hidden near the room's fireplace in the sitting area, and another two in the Cabinet Room. The office's telephones were linked to the system as well. Every phone call and every word spoken during the remainder of the Nixon presidency would be preserved forever (ultimately there would be more than 3,700 hours of tape recordings).[18]

One more drama was unfolding in February 1971. Forty-year-old Rand Corporation analyst Daniel Ellsberg had worked in the Pentagon in the 1960s under defense secretary Robert McNamara. After numerous trips to war-torn Vietnam, Ellsberg contributed to a top-secret report about the government's decision-making regarding the war. He was sickened by the lies about the war's progress even as the body count mounted, and he felt it was time Americans knew the truth. He spent months secretly copying the report's seven thousand pages, then tried to interest anti-war senators in bringing the story to light. They weren't interested, but the *New York Times* was, and published the leaked report, which became known as the Pentagon Papers.[19]

⸺

"A National Cancer Authority will cut through red tape, energize the search for cures, and bring victory by the end of the decade." Mary had recently spoken these words enthusiastically to a journalist, but they angered some at NIH. "My colleagues and I have spent much of our lives trying to move the national research enterprise towards productive results," a senior official was reported to have said. "It makes me mad for Johnny-come-latelies like Benno Schmidt to go around saying we're just a bunch of bureaucrats who are not committed to finding a cure for cancer!"[20]

Now, on March 9, Mary was seated in room 4232 of the New Senate Building, waiting for Senator Kennedy to call to order the first hearings on S. 34. The hearings would cover two days, and testimony this first day would be from those opposed to the bill. Frequently it is the proponents of a bill who speak first. But in flipping that tradition, Kennedy, Mary, and the members of the crusade would have the advantage of seeing their adversaries' cards, and be better able to play their own hand the next day.

Joining Kennedy were five of the thirteen senators on the subcommittee: bill co-sponsor Jacob Javits; Javits's fellow Republican, Peter Dominick of Colorado; and Democrats Thomas Eagleton of Missouri, Alan Cranston of California, and Claiborne Pell of Rhode Island. Kennedy began by outlining the history that had brought them to the hearings, using statistics that Mary had provided. He also informed those present that S. 34 now had fifty-two co-sponsors (Mary and Quinn's hard work had paid off). This was a Senate majority, Kennedy said, and "that fact makes clear the commitment of the Senate to take affirmative action on this matter as quickly as possible." He acknowledged that questions had arisen about the creation of the proposed National Cancer Authority, saying he felt it was necessary, as had the Panel of Consultants, whose members had voted unanimously. "If it is not necessary to create another agency," he said, "and none of us wishes to create additional agencies if they are not required, then the case will have to be clearly and incontrovertibly made by those who hold that view."[21]

The day's witnesses included representatives from the AAMC and the Federation of American Societies for Experimental Biology, along with Dr. Philip Lee, former HEW assistant secretary for health and scientific affairs. Also testifying were administration members Dr. Roger Egeberg (now filling Lee's old position at HEW), NCI's Dr. Baker, NIH's Dr. Marston, and the surgeon general,

Dr. Jesse Steinfeld. The testimony of each witness was nearly entirely directed at debunking the benefit of creating a new agency. Each made the point that the new Cancer Authority wouldn't have the benefit of working with other institutes, which might suddenly find something pertinent to cancer research. That left many wondering whether the institutes would be prohibited from sharing lifesaving discoveries with non-NIH entities. This was certainly not the historical or current practice, as NIH researchers frequently collaborated with scientists at universities and cancer centers.

Equally puzzling were the witnesses' agreements with major points in the panel's report. Of course they should make cancer a national goal. Of course they could create better managerial practices to move things along more quickly. Of course more money should be devoted to research. And all of those things could just as easily be done with NCI remaining intact and in place. But if that was true, Mary wondered, why hadn't they done so long before? Why was the threat of creating a new agency the impetus to finally "declare war on cancer"?

Kennedy didn't spend much time questioning anyone's testimony until it was Baker's turn. "I would like to ask whether we, at the present time, have a comprehensive overall program for the conquest of cancer," the senator said. Baker spoke of "managed plans" and trying continually to "readjust priorities." Kennedy tried again. "I would be interested to know if you have, in any one place, a comprehensive plan to meet the crisis of cancer."[22] The back-and-forth continued in this vein until first Egeberg and then Marston attempted to answer the question. But neither was succinct. It was clear to Kennedy, Mary, and everyone else in the room that the flaw in the administration's position was that they had no real plan to kill the disease that was killing millions.

When Dr. Lee testified, he presented a number of letters, including one from Mary's old adversary Dr. Shannon, former NIH director. Lee explained that the doctor would have been there in person but had just undergone an operation that had reduced his voice to a whisper. His sentiments, however, came through loud and clear. Naturally he, too, was against a separate cancer agency, and was not kind in his reference to Mary: "I predict that orderly governance

would be replaced by anarchy . . . program emphasis would be entirely determined by uncritical zealots, by experts in advertising and pubic relations, and
by rapacious 'empire builders.'"[23] (Those words would also make a big splash in
a *Washington Post* article that would come out the next day.) Lee completed his
testimony shortly before one o'clock, and Kennedy adjourned the subcommittee
until the next morning.

After a lunch break, Mary, Quinn, panel members, and representatives from
ACS met in the hearing room to prepare for the next day. Schmidt had written
a twenty-four-page statement that would be presented on behalf of the panel.
Quinn took on the job of coaching the witnesses, as he had done many times on
behalf of the crusade. When they reassembled at nine-thirty the next day, only
two senators from the subcommittee were present: Kennedy and Javits. They
and the testifying panel members all knew one another, some better than others.
Mary sat in the same seat as she had the day before.

Schmidt presented his statement. Then he called on fellow panel member
Dr. Holland to bring the senators up to date on the recent advancements that
had led them to conclude the time was right for an all-out war on cancer. Holland spoke of the virus research, the successes of chemotherapy and radiation,
and the newly discovered dangers of environmental chemicals.

Dr. Clark was up next, pointing out the need for "a drastic reduction in the
number of people involved in administrative decisions. . . . In the past, when
the Federal Government has desired to give top priority to a major scientific
project of the magnitude of that involved in the conquest of cancer, it has on
occasion . . . given the responsibility for the project to an independent agency."[24]
The parallel between the proposed cancer agency and the AEC and NASA was
crystal clear. Creating a new agency had nothing to do with the level of scientific
knowledge of a given problem. Rather, it had everything to do with layers of
bureaucracy.

The testimony of each of the six panel members present also made clear
why they had been appointed. As she had done at the senators' luncheon, Anna's
words spoke to the human element of S. 34: "My mind goes back to when I was

Assistant Secretary of Defense. I appeared before you and other members of the Senate time and time again to ask for sums so great, that the money we are asking for today for the fight against cancer seems infinitesimal."

She reiterated Mary's figures of the government's per capita expenditures, ending with just 89¢ going to cancer research. "Senators," she concluded, "if we published a casualty list of those who died of cancer as we do of those who die in the war, it would come to almost a thousand people a day. . . . I believe we are asking for too little, and personally I would have asked for more."[25]

Mary had always been amazingly free of pride of authorship. Instead, she placed credit with those whose knowledge or influence enabled them to help her—often, as in this case, against considerable odds. Kennedy, members of the panel, and everyone in the crusade had adopted the same passion for, and ownership of, the Conquest of Cancer Act. And that was just how she liked it. Dr. Holland would later call Mary the most important person in the cancer revolution. That revolution was just beginning.

Chapter 14

"If Someone Isn't Concerned, Nothing Will Ever Get Done"

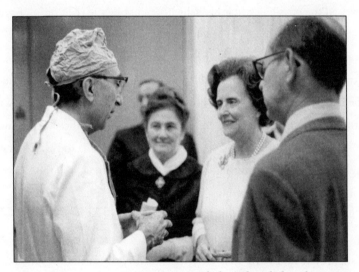

Mary visiting Dr. Michael DeBakey at his hospital, circa 1970s.

"Cancer is not contagious. But the idea that cancer might soon be cured, if enough money is spent, has recently spread among science policy makers like an infectious disease." Robert J. Bazell wrote these words in a March 1971 issue of *Science* magazine. With virtuosic skill he took readers through the individual components of S. 34, explaining that the Laskerites viewed "the current leadership of NIH and NCI, in particular, as lacking the imagination and the pizzazz necessary to hustle for funds in Congress."[1]

Given her ardent desire to fly below the radar, Mary wasn't particularly thrilled to have her name mentioned in the article. But that statement was spot on. As any good journalist should, Bazell then also presented the other side of the coin. Quoting Sol Spiegelman, director of Columbia University's Institute of Cancer Research, on the question of curing the disease: "An all-out effort to cure cancer at this time would be like trying to land a man on the moon without knowing Newton's laws of gravity." There were quotes from James Shannon as well that were, unsurprisingly, negative. But Bazell ended on a high note: "Even if the scientists criticize Mary Lasker's sledge-hammer approach to the subtleties of basic versus applied research, they must face the fact that she gets them more money, and the possibility that her schemes might be the right ones." Bazell was spot on: Mary didn't much care what people thought of her process. Her sole mission was continuing to build the research treasury.

And now Mary had discovered a new battlefront. Nearly three decades earlier she had made her initial (and shocking) call on the American Society for the Control of Cancer. In the intervening years much had changed. The American Cancer Society had been renamed, was far better funded, and was doing more research. Mary just assumed ACS would be strongly in favor of the Conquest of Cancer Act. She assumed wrong.

"They said it was illegal for them to back legislation," Mary huffed incredulously. "Well, I got them a legal opinion. It wasn't illegal. In fact it was their *duty* to be supportive and share that view with their constituents." As the honorary chair of the ACS board, as well as being an active member of the board and the executive committee, she dug a little further. "There were people in the cancer society who did not want large amounts of money spent [on research] by the federal government. They thought that would make it impossible for them to raise money." And that might trickle down to personnel cutbacks, which, she surmised, was their real fear.

From Mary's point of view, the large national ACS network was crucial for spreading the word about S. 34 to the American population. Plus there was another reason to garner their support: many of the top executives of ACS were Republicans. Mary had always sought as much bipartisan support as possible for the crusade, as evidenced by the makeup of the Panel of Consultants. She knew that if the conservative ACS executives supported S. 34, Republican lawmakers would consider it more carefully. The task of swaying those execs fell to the Republican "sugar daddies" of the panel: Bobst, Schmidt, and Rockefeller. Happily, their combined powers of persuasion delivered the crucial prize. On April 3, at the annual Science Writers' Seminar, ACS president Dr. Marvin Pollard announced that the organization absolutely supported the Conquest of Cancer Act, including the need for a separate cancer authority. It would, he said, free the current NCI "of its many layers of bureaucracy which now dilute its priorities and retard its progress."[2] That message of official ACS support was spread to local divisions from coast to coast. Mary breathed a sigh of relief, though that relief would be only temporary.

The U.S. Constitution makes certain that every law can only be enacted after thorough discussion by the legislative branch. Over the course of nearly two hundred years, that process had become extremely complicated. Although Senators Kennedy and Javits first introduced S. 34 on the full Senate floor, it was immediately referred to the Health Subcommittee of the larger Committee on Labor and Public Welfare, as per protocol. The public hearings would be held on March 9 and 10.

A bill is "reported" (or "passed on") by the subcommittee when it has received a majority of aye votes, moving on to the full committee. Along the way, it might be amended ("marked up") or an alternative bill might be proposed. Egos become involved, resulting in senators adding or removing their names as co-sponsors. Amendments mean that new copies of the bill must be created, and prior to the digital world, the entire bill was reprinted every time. The final step—if the bill is not "disposed of," or completely laid to rest—is the Rules Committee, which decides when the bill should go to the full Senate floor for a vote.

This process is duplicated—often simultaneously—in the House. If there are variations in the two bills, a Conference Committee is formed, with members from both legislative chambers meeting to resolve the differences. When everyone is satisfied and the bill passes both chambers, it's signed by the Speaker of the House and the president of the Senate before going to the White House, where it is officially signed into law by the president.

Mary had learned the steps to this arduous and complicated dance over the years. With regard to S. 34, she realized that getting it reported out of the sub-committee was going to be tight. Democrats held a narrow majority, with eight members on the subcommittee to the Republicans' six. Although Democrats were nearly always in favor of bills regarding health, Mary discovered that two of the subcommittee's Democratic senators were violently opposed. And that could tip the majority. It was up to Quinn to discover how and why this had happened.

Dr. Lee, former HEW assistant secretary and now chancellor of the University of California at San Francisco, had gotten the ear of one of California's senators, Alan Cranston. It had been Lee who had presented the negative letters in the March hearings. The other Democratic senator to oppose S. 34 was Gaylord Nelson of Wisconsin, an avid conservationist who was responsible for the establishment of Earth Day (the inaugural celebration had been held the previous year). Nelson had been contacted by a young plant physiologist who was now a professor of enzymology at the University of Wisconsin. Like Lee, the professor was convinced that nothing good could come from changing the sluggish levels of bureaucracy within NIH. He was very persuasive, and Nelson was convinced he was right.

Mary was now haunted by the concerns Kennedy and Humphrey had voiced at the Senate luncheon. The proponents of S. 34 did indeed need big publicity, but not because of the amount of money requested in the bill. Rather, she saw it was the possibility of disrupting the comfortable status quo that had awakened many sleeping giants. And while the references to NASA and the AEC were intended to demonstrate the rationale for setting up an independent National Cancer Authority, there was an earlier model in the government. It was, after all, World War II's Office of Scientific Research and Development and its health component, the Committee on Medical Research, that had gotten Mary thinking about enlarging NIH in the first place.

The time had come to call her friend Eppie Lederer, as she and Alice had discussed at the Greenhouse. Mary told her about the trouble they were in. "I thought unless we had a massive letter-writing campaign directed at senators, we wouldn't get the bill out of the subcommittee," Mary explained. She sent Lederer a copy of S. 34 and the Big Fact Book. That was all the evidence Lederer needed. On April 20, 1971, Ann Landers's fifty-seven million readers (she was syndicated in 750 American newspapers) were treated to a masterly column.

"Dear Readers: If you are looking for a laugh today, you'd better skip Ann Landers. If you want to be part of an effort that might save millions of lives—maybe your own—please stay with me." Astutely pointing out that practically no one reading her column was so lucky as to not have had their lives changed in some way by "this dread disease," Ann said that she supported the creation of the National Cancer Authority, likening it—as others before her had—to the way NASA functioned. She urged her readers to contact their senators, and she finished the column with a passionate plea: "Today you have the opportunity to be a part of the mightiest offensive against a single disease in the history of our country. If enough citizens let their Senators know they want bill S. 34 passed, it will pass. I urge each and every person who reads this column to write to his two Senators at once—or better yet, send telegrams. . . . No one can do everything, but each of us can do something."[3]

Ann's words moved hearts, and more than half a million people did exactly what she asked. Senator Adlai Stevenson III of Illinois (son of Mary's friend) reported that twenty-eight thousand letters arrived at his office. Republican Charles Percy, Illinois's other senator, also received twenty-eight thousand. Senator Fred Harris, a Democrat from Oklahoma with experience in biomedical research as chair of the Government Operations Committee, had opposed the bill, but it was an election year and the groundswell from the column and the letters he received persuaded him to join the ranks of what he called the "mighty offensive." The payoff was that the column's real targets, Cranston and Nelson, each received a whopping sixty thousand letters.[4]

Topping that off, on Sunday, May 2, full-page ads appeared in newspapers across the country. Again, under the aegis of Mary's Citizens Committee for the Conquest of Cancer, the ad carried the text of the Ann Landers column. It also included the names, addresses, and telephone numbers of each state's two senators. Readers were asked to write them, requesting their support for S. 34. The trickle-down from the media coverage of the deluge enhanced the effect even more. Senate staffers, completely overwhelmed by a sea of letters, plopped signs reading "Impeach Ann Landers" on their desks throughout the Senate's office buildings.

"It was a piece of great fortune," Mary said, giving all the credit to her friend, "because without this, we would just never have a chance."

⤳

After his January State of the Union address, reporters had asked Nixon why he was suddenly interested in medicine. He replied it was because his favorite aunt had died of cancer. In truth, it was a quest to stop a Kennedy presidential run. This came through clearly on an Oval Office tape. "I want a lot more use of wiretapping," Nixon said to Haldeman. "Are we doing that? Tailing and so forth? I mean particularly on Teddy. . . . Keep after him [Kennedy], see?"[5]

Not long after that recording, Nixon wrote a memo to Ehrlichman about S. 34: "Ted Kennedy is on a surefire public-relations and political wicket when he comes out for a special approach with a special agency. If we are going to spend the money, the least we can do is to get some credit for having a new approach. We will not get it if we simply put another hundred million dollars in the bowels of NIH and have the program lost forever as far as public view is concerned."[6]

Nixon's obsession became so obvious that a Kennedy staffer chuckled, "You know how the State Department has an Israel desk and a Laos desk? Well, somewhere down there in the White House there's a Kennedy desk, keeping track of everything we do."[7] It was a humorous comparison. It was also, essentially, true.

After that first round of S. 34 hearings, Kennedy had written to HEW secretary Richardson. The subcommittee, he said, was anxious to hear the administration's thoughts about any amendments that might be needed for S. 34. The secretary responded with a four-page plan replete with "mobilize," "emphasize," "expedite," and other verbs describing how the government was going to tackle the conquest of cancer.[8] Their plan, however, just moved agencies around like pieces on a chessboard. But Richardson's letter bought time for Nixon and his administration to decide what they should do. The president's assistant for health affairs, Jim Cavanaugh, was tasked with the job.

Cavanaugh (who had a doctorate in hospital and health administration) had been working for the Nixon White House since the beginning of the administration. On April 26, he circulated a memo lamenting the fact that Kennedy probably already had the subcommittee votes he needed to move S. 34 along. Cavanaugh had gone to the Hill, where he, too, discovered that the argument was not one of money. Rather, "it solely revolves around the question of a separate authority." He further opined that most lawmakers thought it was too late for them to draft a counter-resolution. "If the administration had had a bill of its own two months ago," Cavanaugh wrote, "I think we would be in a very different position than we are today." And then: "Things are about as bad, even worse, on the promotional side of things. . . . The Mary Lasker group ha[s] planned a series of one-half to full page advertisements in major papers."[9]

Four days later, Cavanaugh wrote another memo, this one directed to Ken Cole, Nixon's domestic affairs advisor. He first outlined the problem they faced. "There is an excellent chance that unless we take immediate action, Senator Kennedy will claim and receive credit for your initiative," he wrote, referring to the cancer reference in the State of the Union address. Cavanaugh again wrote that Mary had been the impetus for the entire cancer plan, beginning with the Yarborough Commission and right up to the current Senate bill. She was, Cavanaugh said, "probably Senator Kennedy's greatest ally in the attempt to have the American public believe that Kennedy is the one who is responsible for the cancer initiative." He reiterated that Mary was behind the Ann Landers column and the ensuing newspaper ads. (Perhaps there was also a White House Mary Lasker desk.)

"The Lasker forces are working very heavily," Cavanaugh's memo continued, "to not only secure enactment of the bill but to see that it is Senator Kennedy who receives the credit. . . . Let me stress that the problem is not over the amount of money to be made available for cancer research, but lies in the organizational question of how best to administer the cancer research effort."[10]

To that point, an aggravating question begged to be asked. If cancer was the massively complex problem that the nation's scientists and all the NIH administrators claimed it was, why wouldn't they embrace this aggressive plan to attack and end it?

Cavanaugh's memo listed four options, each with pros and cons. One of the pros always included a statement of how that option would enhance the administration's image (playing to Nixon's ego), while one of the cons always included how the option enhanced Kennedy's image (playing to Nixon's paranoia). The president made his choice just as the subcommittee was preparing to mark up its final version of S. 34.

Although Mary could only guess at what was being done behind closed doors at the White House, she was worried. "Nelson was still against the bill, Cranston was still against it, and the Republicans were against the bill," she fretted. Plus, Democratic senator Walter Mondale was unsure what his vote might be. Without those three Democrats, getting S. 34 out of the subcommittee was looking unlikely. "I realized that we just really didn't have the votes," Mary said.

Mary had supported Nelson's bids for office, and while she wasn't a constituent, they were, after all, both from Wisconsin. Quinn had informed her that there were now two very misguided individuals bending Nelson's ear. In addition to the professor, a staffer in the senator's office had joined the ranks of the naysayers. She was boots on the ground, reinforcing daily the professor's rancor, now including his belief that cancer could never be conquered. The message to Nelson was that cancer should not even be discussed.

Knowing she could be more persuasive in person, Mary decided it was time to enter enemy territory, and she made an appointment to see Nelson. He knew who she was, knew she had donated to him, and agreed to the meeting. But his demeanor shocked her. "When I went to appeal to him for the bill, I could see he was hostile," she said. "He certainly didn't receive me in a way that fitted somebody who had been a contributor to him." The meeting changed nothing.

If she couldn't get the Democrat to change his mind, Mary figured, perhaps she could recruit more Republican support. Hoping Bobst would again be the messenger, she told him on the telephone, "Now, listen, you've been interested in this for twenty-five years." Like Mary, Bobst was also still on the ACS board. "If you could persuade the president to go along, we could make a giant step forward." She knew that when Bobst called Nixon, the president always picked up the phone. This time when Bobst called, he announced he was coming to see the president and spending the night. Nixon's calendar was cleared. At their meeting, Bobst minced no words about S. 34's importance. The president told him that he agreed 100 percent. He would pass the word: the bill was to receive the administration's full support.

A week later, the crusade celebrated when they learned that the president would release a statement on May 11. "The time has now come to put our money where our hopes are," Nixon said. He referred again to splitting the atom and landing on the moon, finishing with, "Now we need to apply those same capacities to the conquest of cancer." But he wasn't supporting S. 34; he had a new plan, called the Cancer Cure Program. After the official statement, a reporter asked the president why he was introducing what appeared to be a duplicate of the program currently being considered in the Senate. Nixon was happy to field that question. "I have asked for this because . . . I believe presidential interest and presidential guidance will hasten the cure for cancer."[11] Translation: Kennedy might be able to propose a lot of things, but he could not refer to himself as president.

On the Senate floor, nearly simultaneously with the White House statement, the ranking member of the Subcommittee on Health, Colorado Republican Peter Dominick, introduced S. 1828. In his comments, Dominick said his bill included the same research funding amounts as S. 34, along with its other elements. The only difference was that the cancer research agency would not move out of NIH. This made the scientific community and the AMA happy. Nixon was satisfied, too. He was back in the headlines, having regained the reins of the national cancer program. To all of this, Ann Landers quipped, "When he figured out he couldn't beat us, he joined us!"[12]

However, when Quinn and ACS executive Alan Davis analyzed S. 1828 a few days later, they found discrepancies. The bill made no reference to the president appointing the director of the new agency, or that the director would report only to the president, or that the research budget would be directly approved by the president. In fact, Quinn realized, the bill didn't even remotely resemble what Nixon had outlined in his statement a few days earlier. The administration was saying one thing but doing another. He passed his discovery along to Mary and Schmidt.[13]

Schmidt was livid, and became even more so when a *New York Times* editorial came out against S. 34. He was so apoplectic that he flew from New York to Washington to see Kennedy, sat the senator and his staff director, Leroy Goldman, down, and proceeded to read them the letter he was about to send to the *Times*.

Bobst, however, was unaware of Quinn's findings. He thought that Nixon had made good on his word. He was so thrilled that his friend the president was embracing the panel's recommendations that he called ACS executive vice president Lane Adams to express pride at the president's bold step. By this time, however, Adams also knew about S. 1828's discrepancies. He and Davis discussed it, and realized they had to tell Bobst the truth, and in person. So off they went to his office across town. Once Bobst heard why they'd come, he, too, was furious and called Ken Cole.

"Ken, my friends from the American Cancer Society tell me that the bill that has been introduced hardly resembles what the president told the American people in his press statement a few days ago. . . . I want that changed. I had a clear, concise understanding with the president. It certainly does not help the president to be telling the people one thing and [having] his aides saying another. Please get that corrected."[14] The White House immediately dispatched Cole to New York to meet with Schmidt.

∾

Mary had received reports from both Quinn and Gorman mentioning Jim Cavanaugh as a major player in the Nixon cancer plan. Mary knew who he was, always making it a point to know not just presidents and legislators but staff members as well. Since much of the crusade's success had come from finding friends in unlikely places (such as the Republican Party) it was time to call on Cavanaugh, and they arranged a meeting.

When she arrived at the West Wing, Cavanaugh's secretary escorted her to his office. Cavanaugh thanked Mary for coming and told her the administration was looking forward to her thoughts and recommendations on the cancer research program. Mary looked around his office, smiled at him warmly, and said, "This is only the second time that I've been in a Republican White House." (The first time had been over a year earlier, for the Andrew Wyeth exhibition. But to Mary it seemed more like a decade.)

That icebreaker led to one from Cavanaugh. He told her jovially that the latest cancer incidence data appeared to show that Republicans and Democrats were equally affected by the disease. The president's interest, he said, was finding cures for all Americans. Mary thought that was a good start, and the meeting followed along the same lines. She explained that her interest in conquering cancer had come from those she had lost to the disease, including Albert. She ended with, "If someone isn't concerned, nothing will ever get done." This prompted Cavanaugh to commend the work of the Panel of Consultants, and the meeting came to a friendly close.[15]

Then Mary had another idea. Given that the administration had sent Cole to see Schmidt after Bobst's call, it seemed that the White House considered Schmidt to be the de facto representative of Kennedy, Mary, and the crusade. Perhaps it was time for him to visit Cavanaugh as well. Schmidt was convinced that the success of S. 34 was vital to humanity, and so he agreed without hesitation. He made numerous trips to Washington, D.C., over the ensuing weeks, meeting with Cavanaugh and with Leroy Goldman, too.

In Washington, what goes on behind the scenes is vastly more important (and more interesting) than what goes on out in the open. The two bills now before the Senate had made the major players' motivations clear. The president wanted reelection. Kennedy wanted political redemption. Mary Lasker just wanted to cure cancer.

The conflicting motivations meant that there was one more hurdle to be overcome. On his last visit with Cavanaugh, Schmidt had learned that while Nixon wanted a cancer bill, there was an insurmountable problem. S. 34 had been introduced by Kennedy; he was the subcommittee chairman, and the bill would bear his name. Richard Nixon had made it clear to his staff that he would *never* endorse or sign any bill bearing Ted Kennedy's name. And he would *never* allow Ted Kennedy to receive credit for a cancer bill. Mary couldn't believe she was hearing correctly—that the goal of saving millions of lives was so easily re-placed with political ambition. The only way to now save her crusade was to call Kennedy and ask him for the ultimate favor.

⚞

On June 9, a private meeting was held in a small room of the Old Senate Office Building. Senators Kennedy and Dominick were there, along with various mem-bers of their staffs. Pleasantries were exchanged, and then Kennedy astounded them all by saying to Dominick, "Peter, why don't we report S. 1828." Cancer was the focus, Kennedy reminded his colleague. "Forget my bill. We'll report the president's bill. . . . And Peter, why don't you report it." No one made a sound. Kennedy continued, "I have an amendment to offer . . . strike all [the language] after the enacting clause and substitute in lieu thereof the text of S. 34."[16]

Aside from the name of the act, the enacting clause was identical for every bill ever presented in the halls of Congress. In the case of S. 1828, it read, "Be it enacted by the Senate and House of Representatives of the United States of America in Congress assembled, that this Act may be cited as the 'Act to Conquer Cancer.'" Everything that followed, according to Kennedy's suggested amendment, would be the verbiage from S. 34. While this was an extraordinary gesture of political generosity, it was also politically shrewd. In one fell swoop, Kennedy gave President Nixon the credit for a cancer bill but saw to it that the meat of the bill was based on the recommendations of Mary's Panel of Consul-tants. The cancer institute would be completely autonomous, answering only to the president. Leroy Goldman, who also served as the subcommittee staff counsel, aptly explained later, "We breathed life into the president's bill, using scissors and scotch tape."[17]

⌒

"The American people are demanding action on the cancer front," Senator Kennedy said when he asked the subcommittee to come to order on the morning of June 10. "Forty-five times as many Americans have succumbed to cancer over the last six years than have died in the tragically misguided Indochina war. If progress is not made, one out of every four Americans alive today will contract cancer. And two-thirds of them will die."[18]

Unlike the March hearings, on this day the fourth-floor hearing room in the Old Senate Office Building was crowded with participants and press. In addition to Kennedy, Senators Nelson, Cranston, Eagleton, Javits, and Dominick were on hand for the hearing. So were HEW secretary Richardson and NIH director Marston. The Panel of Consultants would be represented by Schmidt, Farber, and Lee. Mary was seated in the audience, appearing calm and elegant. Her stomach, however, was churning. Kennedy explained for the record that S. 1828 had been introduced on behalf of the administration, and that the administration had requested that the subcommittee hold off on marking up S. 34 until the new bill could be discussed. The subcommittee, Kennedy said, had been happy to do so.

Very few in the room knew about the private meeting that had taken place the day before. When Mary had spoken to Kennedy and he agreed to step back, he explained that Javits's name would also have to be removed from the bill, since they had been the original co-sponsors. They both agreed that Schmidt, a fellow Republican, should break the news to Javits, who absolutely refused to agree to the plan; he would not, under any circumstances, strip Kennedy of the credit he so richly deserved. Schmidt attempted to calm him. "Jack, you don't understand. Ted has taken his name off," asserting that he would not leave until Javits agreed. He finally did.[19]

As soon as Kennedy finished his opening remarks, Javits immediately asked for the floor "to call attention to the really extraordinary exercise of statesmanship by the administration and by the chair. . . . And we also owe a debt in that regard to Senator Dominick."

"Would the chair yield?" Dominick asked when Javits had finished his remarks. He, too, began by gushing, "I, also, want to congratulate the chairman for holding these hearings and for his efforts to work out a mutually agreeable bill with the administration."

Kennedy thanked them both and quipped, "Maybe we ought to just recess the hearing and pass the bill as long as we have everything on track." Laughter echoed through the room. One person, however, did not laugh.[20]

Gaylord Nelson knew all about the private Kennedy-Dominick meeting. The next day Nelson would sputter, "The bill [S. 1828] is S. 34 with insignificant amendments," and then spill the details to the press.[21] But now, in the hearing room, the agenda called for Richardson to begin his testimony.

"As preliminary remarks of members of the committee have emphasized," Richardson said, "there is broad agreement on the very high priority to be attached to mobilizing resources for exploitation and potential breakthroughs in the field of cancer." When Richardson's opening statement was completed, Kennedy questioned him, followed by Javits. Did the secretary think that an independent agency within NIH, headed by a director appointed by the president, could be successful? Richardson said he thought so. Javits then asked if he and Dr. Marston would not only carry out the bill as it was written but also have their hearts in it. Richardson vowed, "I think we can firmly pledge that we would exert our utmost efforts to that end."[22]

Senator Nelson—appearing as agitated as he had been when Mary saw him a few weeks earlier—wanted the floor next. Despite having been an original co-sponsor of S. 34, he said, he had changed his mind after "studying the bill in great depth." He began to question Richardson, but in light of what he knew about the private Kennedy-Dominick meeting, he became angrily confused about which version of S. 1828 the secretary was referring to. Richardson said he was unaware of multiple versions. (No one from HEW had been included in the private meeting.) What ensued, then, was something akin to Abbott and

Costello's "Who's on First," played out for five minutes, as Nelson and Richardson went around in circles about which version of S. 1828 was being discussed.[23]

Nelson's greatest attack, however, was directed to the panel itself. Schmidt, Clark, and Farber testified, reiterating how and why they had arrived at their recommendations. Nelson stated that the panel vote to remove NCI from NIH had been 16–10. Now, he said, three members who had voted yes were having second thoughts, making it a tie. Schmidt explained that everything the panel had agreed to had been by unanimous vote and it was. There were twenty-six members, but not all were present when they voted. When Nelson said that Dr. Joshua Lederberg was the one complaining, Schmidt replied that Lederberg never participated in the panel deliberations or their final vote. Nelson shot back, "Perhaps we misunderstood the two panel members who indicated differently on that issue."[24] There were clearly agitators on the panel. But even with the opposition's letters of support, Nelson's accusation went nowhere, and Kennedy adjourned the hearing at one o'clock.

⁓

On June 12, 1971 (two days after Kennedy and Dominick had shaken hands on S. 1828), Tricia Nixon married Edward Cox in the White House Rose Garden. As the president reviewed the press coverage the next day, it occurred to him that more was needed, and he called Ron Ziegler, his press secretary. The wedding had been carried by the networks, he told Ziegler. Why not suggest it be replayed in prime time during the upcoming week? "Women all want to see the damn thing. If it were the Kennedys it would be rerun every night for three weeks."

Nixon's positive mood changed drastically when his deputy assistant for national security affairs, General Alexander Haig, telephoned a little after noon to talk about a series of *New York Times* articles that would be appearing shortly. The president was unaware of this, and Haig went on to describe the "devastating security breach of the greatest magnitude." Daniel Ellsberg had proceeded with his plan to publicize the Pentagon Papers. The *Times* recognized the bombshell Ellsberg was offering, and had scheduled installments to be run over the next ten days. The material clearly showed the military mismanagement, directed by Presidents Kennedy and Johnson. But more than the meat of the exposé, Nixon was furious that it had been leaked at all.

"Goddamn it! Somebody's got to go to jail!" Nixon told Haldeman later. "It's a conspiracy, Bob. We're going to fight with everything we've got."[25]

The U.S. Justice Department slapped the *Times* with a restraining order, but the Supreme Court ultimately ruled against it. "Only a free and unrestrained press can effectively expose deception in government," Justice Hugo Black wrote.[26] Nixon soon realized the potential political power of the Pentagon Papers (which he preferred to call the McNamara Papers). They contained information about JFK having aided and abetted the assassination of South Vietnam's president Ngo Dinh Diem in 1963. In Nixon's mind, obsessed with enemies—who included Democrats, Congress, the press, the establishment, and the elites—that information could cast a dark shadow over Ted Kennedy's potential presidential run. Ironically, it was those very "enemies" who had just seen to it that Nixon received full credit for launching the war on cancer.

⌇

The day before the subcommittee considered S. 1828, Mary received the Alfred P. Sloan Award from the American Cancer Society. Sloan had been a founder of General Motors and a great philanthropist, and he was the namesake of New York's Sloan Kettering Hospital. It was truly a great honor, made even more exciting when LBJ and Lady Bird surprised Mary at the $100-a-plate dinner to raise funds for ACS. LBJ bestowed the award, telling the fourteen hundred in attendance, "I can't think of a higher national priority than the conquest of cancer and I can't think of a person more likely to do it than Mary Lasker."[27] He was right, of course, but that work would face its next test when the full Senate voted on S. 1828, just twenty-seven days away.

Wednesday, July 7, was a sultry summer day in Washington, D.C., with temperatures and humidity both in the eighties. Despite the air-conditioning in the Senate chamber, the afternoon air was thick up in the gallery where Mary and others associated with the crusade anxiously awaited the proceedings. The eighty senators present that day returned from their recess at three o'clock and were called to order. Over the next two and a half hours, a debate ensued, with Senators Cranston and Nelson still digging in their heels regarding an independent cancer agency. "I am debating the question today," Nelson said, "not in the expectation that I will persuade anybody to change the bill, because I know I will not, on this side. But I am hopeful that the House will give it a deliberate, careful look and will remedy what I think is a serious defect in an otherwise very fine bill."

Nelson continued, "Creating a separate independent institute . . . is going to establish a precedent. . . . In fact, the National Heart and Lung Institute has now requested that they be treated in the same fashion. . . . Their case will be just as good as a case for a separate cancer institute outside of NIH. In fact, the statistics are that 38.4 percent of the people who die in this country die from diseases of the heart. Malignant neoplasms [cancer] cause 16.9 percent of the deaths."[28]

The arguments wore on, until at last Cranston capitulated. "However, we must conquer cancer," Cranston acknowledged. "This measure—considered with care by so many public officials and private citizens . . . like the indomitable Mary Lasker, with the deepest dedication and concern, and with truly remarkable experience in what it takes to launch a vital new undertaking. . . . As a start toward the end of cancer, I, therefore, urge support of this measure."[29]

At five-thirty a vote was called. Seventy-nine senators voted aye, with Nelson standing fast and voting nay. It was one of the most thrilling days in Mary's life as a citizen lobbyist. She had seen to fruition an agreement between two violently opposed sides, an agreement that could quite possibly play a role in erasing the scourge of cancer from the face of the planet. But in doing so, Mary had made a new adversary. His name was Paul Rogers.

Chapter 15

~

"Putting It on the Shelf"

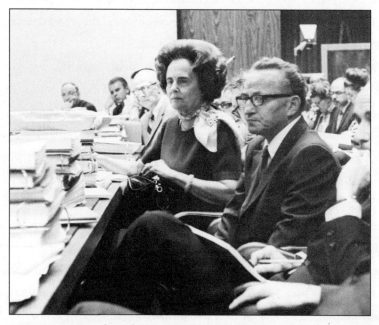

Mary at a hearing for the Conquest of Cancer Act, next to Dr. Sol Spiegelman, circa 1971.

With his wife and three sons in tow, attorney Dwight Rogers left tiny Ocilla, Georgia (population 2,000), in 1925. Settling in Fort Lauderdale, Rogers spent eight years in the Florida House of Representatives and then became a U.S. congressman in 1945. On December 1, 1954, after a round of golf, he was the featured speaker at an evening event at Fort Lauderdale's Bahia Mar Yacht Club. When he finished his speech, he told his dinner companion he wasn't feeling well. Taken first to a nearby doctor,

Rogers was ultimately rushed to the hospital, where he died a few hours later, having suffered a heart attack.[1]

Rogers's middle son, Paul, was practicing law in New York City at the time. But that soon changed. Promising to carry on his father's legacy, the younger Rogers won a special election for his father's House seat on January 11, 1955. He had won eight more elections by January 1971, with thirteen years on the Subcommittee on Public Health and Environment. The subcommittee chairman wasn't terribly interested in its work, and Rogers had happily—albeit unofficially—filled in over the years.[2] When the Democratic caucus voted to limit the number of subcommittees representatives could lead, new chairmanships became available, including that of Public Health and Environment.

At the start of the year, this bit of minutiae didn't seem relevant to Mary and the crusade. Paul Rogers was just another member of the subcommittee. The crusade had always focused on the appropriations committees in Congress. Plus the chair of the subcommittee's powerful parent committee, the Committee on Interstate and Foreign Commerce, was an old friend of Mary's, West Virginia Democrat Harley Staggers. He seemed the more important House connection.

Staggers was committed to the crusade, he assured Mary. After all, a fellow West Virginian had been the originator of the idea to create a National Cancer Institute in 1928. The disease had been, Staggers told her, the very thing "that my friend, Matt Neely, died of. [He tried] to get a cancer bill for years and nothing was ever done." Staggers promised to change that, and announced. personal support for S. 34 when it was initially introduced. In February, along with Mary's other old friend Claude Pepper (who had returned to Congress as a representative in 1963), Staggers introduced a bill with language identical to the Senate's. Quinn had garnered 103 co-sponsors for it. It appeared that with clear skies and fair winds in the House, the cancer bill would sail through with ease.

But Mary wasn't convinced; she was concerned about the vacant subcommittee chairmanship and went to see Staggers. "Listen," she told him emphatically, "[don't] appoint Rogers. He's against this bill, and it's going to be the best thing that could ever happen in the field of cancer." Staggers told Mary she was worrying unnecessarily. He would personally see to it that Rogers would embrace the legislation. Yet as she had feared, four days before the start of the March Senate hearings on S. 34, Rogers became chair of the Public Health and Environment Subcommittee. It was more or less by default: none of his senior colleagues wanted the position, and Rogers wanted it desperately. Soon the tremors from his appointment began to dramatically shake the crusade.

Five years earlier, again with an absent chairman, Rogers had led an extensive investigation into all the health activities of HEW (the parent agency of NIH). Rogers called HEW a "federal maze," saying it "doesn't quite handle all the health matters we thought it did."[3] Yet the twenty-five pages of the report that were devoted to NIH had contained no disparaging comments. And now he was claiming, as so many had, that removing cancer research from NIH would "increase administrative costs, disrupt ongoing work, and set a precedent for other health groups, like heart disease."[4]

Mary couldn't understand why Rogers was defending NIH. "[They were] getting basic information together and putting it on the shelf," she proclaimed. Meanwhile, "everybody in the Senate took it for granted that [they were] doing the maximum to conquer every disease that they were appropriating money for." And so did Rogers; he had no reason to think otherwise.

Given his new position as chairman of the subcommittee that would hold the first set of hearings on a House cancer bill, Rogers assumed Mary and her forces would pay him a call shortly after he assumed the chair. But no one came. It was a mistake Mary would deeply regret.

~

"There are 17 types of cancer on which 37 drugs show transient regressions," Mary had pointed out in 1970. Chemotherapy was certainly the future in cancer treatment; Sidney Farber and others were proving just that, with their continued success in combating childhood leukemia and other forms of cancer. Although oncology was still a new, low-prestige specialty in medicine, Mary was convinced that victory was at hand. "When you get to this stage you realize that it's really money, experience, determination and making a goal of the conquest that will finally do it." She felt it was a two-pronged attack: work toward curing cancer with drugs and also toward preventing it with vaccinations.

"People interested in virology are already talking about a vaccine against leukemia by 1973," she explained. "And they also talk of the possibility of a particle or genetic element that's built into everyone. Under stress, it might be triggered and could possibly cause cancer." Even a small breakthrough in those areas would go a long way to persuade the legislators to pass the Conquest of Cancer bill in the House as the Senate had. She was a positive thinker, but she also planned ahead. The cancer bill would need money appropriated to it.

Mary's interest in virology—and its research at NCI—made her familiar with the names of those working in the field. One of these was Dr. Robert Gallo, who had arrived at NCI in 1965, at the age of twenty-eight. By 1971, he was deeply involved in virus research. Then one day he received a call from Mary. She wanted him to accompany her to a meeting with Representative William Natcher, a member of the House Subcommittee on Labor, Health, Education, and Welfare Appropriations. Gallo was stunned, telling his supervisor, Dr. Vincent DeVita, that he thought it was a little weird. "What will I say?" Gallo asked. DeVita replied, "Bob, you do what Mary Lasker says."

Riding with him in her car to the Capitol, Mary told Gallo exactly what to say: emphasize the positives in cancer virus research, tell Natcher what was coming out of NCI, and talk about the progress on a cancer vaccine. Gallo was nervous and said, "Mrs. Lasker, cancer is complicated with many implications." "Just emphasize the positive," she told him breezily. He evidently did such a good job that he was next invited to one of Mary and Deeda Blair's famous—and strategic—dinner parties. On this particular occasion, one of the guests was the beautiful actress Jennifer Jones. (Several decades earlier, she had won an Academy Award for her starring role in *The Song of Bernadette*, and gone on to marry the producer, David O. Selznick.)

The actress arrived at the Blairs' wearing a backless dress, accenting her broad shoulders and tiny waist. A starstruck Gallo followed her down to the lower-level terrace, where the dinner would take place. The formula for these events never varied. Those with the power to act mingled with those possessing ideas for action, all topped off with the glamour of Hollywood. Tables for four were set, and at each sat a celebrity (thrilled with the guests' attention), a journalist (seeking a scoop from the celebrity), a politician (hoping the journalist would publicize recent successes), and a scientist (told to cater only to the important person at their table, the politician). Gallo was shocked to discover he was seated at Jones's table. With difficulty, he focused on his task: making virology sound as exciting as possible to Senator Mark Hatfield, chair of the Senate Appropriations Committee.[5]

Not long afterward, on Thursday, July 15, Mary had her first meeting with Representative Rogers. Accompanying her for lunch were Dr. Farber and Indiana representative John Brademas. Although Brademas had little to do with health legislation, he was a Mary Lasker ally and an art devotee. That made Mary a devotee of his as well. They hadn't been seated in the House restaurant for very long when Rogers politely informed his tablemates that making NCI independent would violate the integrity of NIH and possibly that of medical research. Though he listened respectfully, he remained resolute.

Rogers knew full well that the House was keen to work with the Senate so that the cancer legislation could be sent to the president. When Senator Dominick introduced his original bill, Rogers had introduced his own, nearly identical version in the House. But his willingness to cooperate vanished when Dominick's revised bill used Kennedy's language, which Rogers vehemently opposed. He was further irritated when an article came out quoting Gorman, who suggested that Rogers would have to come around since Staggers was in favor of the Kennedy proposal, "and chairmen," Gorman asserted in a veiled threat, "are powerful men." Gorman made a similar indelicate assertion a month later. The two statements infuriated Quinn; Gorman, Quinn told Mary, needed to keep his nose out of the cancer world.[6]

Rogers also disliked the reference to Kennedy as "Mr. Health." The two men had been chairmen of their respective subcommittees for nearly the same amount of time, but Rogers had been on his much longer and felt he held seniority in health legislation. Therefore, he thought, he had far more claim to be Congress's "Mr. Health."[7]

The least emotional of the reasons for Rogers's recalcitrance was the solidest one. As the subcommittee's new chairman, Rogers needed to prove his mettle. He was not about to be swept away on the tide of public thrill over a cure for cancer. Nor would he be railroaded by any health lobby, regardless of its power and sophistication.

Lunch ended as it had been conducted: politely and with restraint. Rogers informed Mary that there were going to be hearings, long hearings, with no stone left unturned. It seemed as though the two of them had absolutely nothing in common other than being Democrats. But beneath their differences there was, in fact, something that might have softened their relationship considerably. Each, at the age of thirty-three, had experienced the sudden death of their father. Both had been in New York City at the time of the deaths, and both had had to make long journeys to get home to their mothers. Sadly, that commonality never came to the fore.

Not long after that lunch, Rogers made it known that he would not immediately be holding hearings on the cancer bill; there were other items taking precedence. Mary was now afraid the cancer act wouldn't make it into law before year's end. The congressional summer recess would begin at the close of business on Friday, August 6, and legislators wouldn't return until mid-September. The Vietnam War and other issues would distract them, and cancer would once again be swept aside. She appealed directly to Staggers, who told her, "If he [Rogers] doesn't go along I'll hold the hearings myself." She and the other members of the crusade thought that was a very brave promise, as it would have been a total breach of protocol for a full committee chairman to usurp the duties of a subcommittee chair. However, the promise was comforting, and so Mary prepared for her summer sojourn.

⁓

One key to Mary's success in health lobbying was her visibility. Money could buy visibility, to be sure, but the *type* of visibility is also key. Everyone knew her, and those who took the time to really get to know her found her passion for the health of Americans inspiring. Visibility, however, is something one must work at; it can vanish like smoke through a keyhole.

On July 25, Mary headed to Paris aboard a Braniff Airlines 747. (In six weeks she would be elected to the airline's board of directors, one of only a scant few women who served on major corporate boards at the time.) With first class marketed as "a place to live well in flight," this trip was shorter than her previous ship crossings but no less glamorous. With Deeda Blair as her companion, Mary's first stop in Paris, as always, was the couture fashion shows, before heading for the Riviera and La Fiorentina. The season's calendar began with a party for Lady Bird Johnson. But it was one of the last events at the end of the season that would start all the tongues wagging. Under a balmy night sky, adorned with a full moon and an array of stars, everyone who was anyone was invited to the Red and White Ball.

The ninety-year-old Hôtel du Cap at the isolated point of Cap d'Antibes was the location for the September 3 ball, and—as with Truman Capote's ball in 1966—there were very specific attire instructions: women were to wear either red or white (or a combination), and men were to wear white tuxes or white dinner jackets. Host Earl Blackwell had selected the colors because of the availability of red and white flowers for decor, and because they were the colors of Monaco's flag (Blackwell hoped to entice Prince Rainier and Princess Grace to come, but they sent their regrets ahead of time).[8]

Mary and her houseguests, the Blairs and the Van der Kamps (he was still the curator at Versailles), traveled the fifty miles of Riviera coastline from La Fiorentina in her limousine. On arrival, they were directed to the hotel's open-air pavilion, sandwiched between the immense swimming pool and the Mediterranean Sea. The four hundred guests grazed at two buffets and danced, all while downing copious amounts of champagne. The night was capped off with a spectacular display of red and white fireworks.

Two days later, Mary received a cable from Schmidt. The word in Congress was that Rogers intended to begin hearings very soon, certainly by September 15. Although she had planned to stay a few more weeks, Mary arrived back in New York on the eleventh and headed immediately for Washington, D.C. For better or worse, the climax of her decades of work was about to unfold.

She scheduled a meeting with Rogers on September 13. "I'll give testimony to you privately," Mary told him on the telephone. She brought him a summary showing that over the past twenty years, NIH hadn't brought about any change in the nation's death rate. She pointed out that to change the death rate, there must be some movement in addressing the major causes, cancer and heart disease. But that hadn't happened. She showed him a list of what NIH had accomplished, and while some of those accomplishments might make an impact over the next decade or so, they were not making an immediate difference in helping the population live longer *today*. Rogers was again very courteous. However, he wasn't moved.

The next day, Rogers phoned Mary at the Blairs' home. A package was on its way to her. "It's my bill," he told her, "and I think that you'll like it." She already knew that his bill had been highly influenced by the Association of American Medical Colleges, and this was not good news. "The deans of medical colleges are not in the least anxious to do anything," Mary later observed. "Deans aren't interested in curing conditions, just basic science. They don't care whether anything is solved or not, as long as they have money to keep the medical schools going." Mary certainly wasn't on this crusade just to please deans.

She tore open Rogers's package as soon as it arrived. The bill contained little that was useful, nor did it much resemble the Senate bill. He had, however, added $20 million for control grants (to fund clinical trials), which had previously been eliminated by NIH. In addition, grants of up to $5 million would be available for cancer centers. Both of those things pleased her; but the organizational restructuring for cancer research was glaringly missing.

Hearing room 2318 of the Rayburn House Office Building was packed when Chairman Rogers called the subcommittee to order at one o'clock on Wednesday, September 15. Mary sat in the first row of the gallery, so visible that Staggers waved at her as he took his chair in the long row of House member seats at the front of the room. Between them and the gallery, a table with microphones awaited those who would testify.

"The Subcommittee on Public Health and Environment is beginning hearings today on several proposed bills, all of which have as their common aim the development of a cure for cancer," Rogers began. "This committee intends to closely investigate all proposals and to listen with open minds to additional comment from the list of witnesses who will come before us in the coming weeks. We intend to thoroughly examine all alternatives which will result in legislation which will bring us to our goal in the shortest time possible."[9]

Rogers's hearings, however, would not be short. Like a well-trained draft horse, he planned to plod along, as opposed to the Senate hearings' quick race to the finish line. He told the assembled group that the hearings would span three weeks, as opposed to the Senate's three days. The chairman next listed the plethora of bills that had already been introduced to the House on the subject of "a cure for cancer," including his own, H.R. 10681. As Mary had observed, Rogers's bill—the National Cancer Attack Act—differed from S. 1828 in some very crucial ways. First, its scope had been broadened to include other killer diseases and institutes. The directors of those institutes would be raised to the level of the NIH director, and all would be presidential appointees. However, none of those directors would report directly to the president; the layers of bureaucracy would remain. And the National Cancer Institute would remain within NIH.

At the table were seated that day's witnesses, who included NIH director Marston, HEW secretary Richardson, and his new assistant secretary, Dr. Merlin DuVal, who had replaced Dr. Egeberg. (In the spring, Egeberg had complained, "The White House just doesn't know what is going on in the health field. I just can't get through to Ehrlichman. I may be fired because of my words and actions, but I won't quit." A short time later he admitted, "I don't want the whole job anymore," and left.)[10] Sitting behind them, also in the front row of the gallery, was NCI director Baker. As was expected, the majority of the congressmen's questions revolved around S. 1828 and removing NCI from NIH.

At times, the questioning was rapid-fire, with congressmen trying to confuse the witnesses. At the end of the afternoon, the ranking member, Minnesota Republican Ancher Nelsen, made an interesting observation. Likening the case before them to others he had been involved in, he pointed out, "Many of the things we have talked about today, in similar cases, were worked out. Sometimes this is best done in not too much of a forum, but rather in a quiet way. So I may say to my good chairman of the subcommittee, 'The proud young fathers take it from a grandfather, don't get so excited. We will work it all out.'"

Rogers snapped back, "We have to get excited, Mr. Nelsen, and get some action. That is what we are going to do."[11] The chairman had no interest in sitting idly by. Nor had he been idle during the summer. While Mary was in Europe, Rogers had been in contact with his subcommittee members, sending them articles disparaging S. 1828. He had also had an unlikely visitor. Democratic representative J. J. Pickle had advised Benno Schmidt to get to know Rogers and to keep the pressure on him, which Schmidt did over several meetings. But Rogers never wavered.

As he called the second day of hearings to order at ten the next morning, Chairman Rogers said, "We are very pleased today to have a most distinguished witness . . . Senator Gaylord Nelson. He has been most active in this field. . . . [T]he committee welcomes you, Senator Nelson. We invite you to take the stand."[12]

Nelson reiterated all the same arguments he had made in the Senate: removing NCI from NIH would be the demise of the research agency; other institutes would want equal treatment; there was no evidence of organizational problems. The last of those claims was particularly puzzling, since NCI director Baker had given ample examples of just that in a hearing the previous year.

Nelsen then questioned Nelson, asking about the tally of the Senate vote on S. 1828. Seventy-nine to one, Nelson told him, and affirmed proudly that he was the lone holdout. "The thing that concerns me," the congressman told the senator, "is that I detect a little bit of guarding of present muscle in the program by competing groups that I think is very unfortunate. I think there is great merit to what you say, and I think there is great merit to the observation of the objective, and I hope we can work this thing out as we have done with . . . many other endeavors and by sitting down together."[13]

Next to present testimony was New York representative John J. Rooney. He described himself as a "competent witness" because he had been successfully treated for lung cancer in 1966. He had been a good friend of Representative Fogarty's, and he testified brilliantly. His remarks, however, probably gained their eloquence as a result of the news Mary had shared earlier: their mutual friend Lukė Quinn had been hospitalized on the NIH campus after it was discovered that his cancer had metastasized to his liver.

Claude Pepper was up next, reminding the assembled group that he had been a co-sponsor of the 1937 bill that had created the National Cancer Institute. "We went along without any increase in the amount of money available for that Institute until about 1940, and due to the initiative of one of the greatest ladies this country has every known, one of the loveliest, Mrs. Albert Lasker, who is in the room today."[14] (His words were kind, if not a little embarrassing to Mary.) Pepper continued that her initiative, along with that of Albert, had inspired the Senate to increase the institute's appropriations. What was being asked for, Pepper said, was by no means out of the question. Congress had never been consulted about the $2 billion spent on the atomic bomb, nor on the still undisclosed amount for the moon landing.

After a recess, the hearings began again three days later, on Monday, September 20. Now it was the crusade's turn to be heard. Testimonies prepared, panel members Schmidt, Farber, Clark, Holland, Krim, and Scott sat at the witness table. As he had done when testifying before the Senate, Schmidt explained the panel's three main goals in the effort to conquer cancer: an effective organization, a comprehensive plan, and adequate funding. He then asked his colleagues to elaborate.

The doctors all made impressive and compelling cases. Scott's was particularly pertinent, since the renowned radiologist had been treated for cancer while working on the panel. (He would succumb to a return of the disease in less than a year.)

Farber then had one more point to make: "We cannot wait for full understanding; the 325,000 patients with cancer who are going to die this year cannot wait; nor is it necessary. . . . The history of medicine is replete with examples of cures obtained years, decades and even centuries before the mechanism of action was understood for these cures."[15] Aside from his work, he, too, had a personal connection to the disease. Unbeknownst to anyone in the room (and very few outside of his immediate family), he had been diagnosed with colorectal cancer and had undergone a colostomy.

Again and again, the congressmen opposed to creating a separate cancer agency proclaimed it would be the ruination of NIH. The director of the National Heart and Lung Institute had gone on record saying he supported S. 1828, particularly as it might apply to his institute down the road. That might have been perceived as a victory for the bill's opponents, but it made no more sense to Mary than did the argument that S. 1828 might displease medical school deans. Her goal was to cure cancer at the earliest opportunity. Why did it seem the room was filled with those resistant to that idea?

Maine Democrat Peter Kyros was up next to question the panel members. He referred to Senator Nelson's accusation that the panel had not had a unanimous vote on its recommendations, and he asked whether the vote to take NCI out of NIH had not actually been 16–10. Schmidt again explained (as he had to Nelson himself) that while it was true there were twenty-six members on the panel, four of those members had never come to a single meeting; therefore, that vote count would have been impossible. To those present for the vote, Schmidt said he had read each recommendation aloud, giving the group time to oppose them. No one objected. He had even gone a step farther, contacting those who hadn't attended the meetings and asking if they wished their names removed from the final report. No one responded. Further, Schmitt said, Senator Nelson was neither at a February luncheon to explain their work (the one Mary had hosted) nor at the Senate hearings in March.[16]

One theme that repeated itself throughout the first three days was the "overwhelming number" of medical and scientific organizations, like the AMA and the AAMC, that were opposed to moving NCI. Of course, this wasn't the first time the crusade had butted heads with the AMA.

Schmidt had finally had enough. "I think a vast majority of those of whom you speak are not cancer scientists," he said, "and I would suspect the intuitive response of people who are not cancer scientists to be that this gives cancer a priority." He continued, "The crux of the matter, is whether you want the head of the NIH to run this program or you want the head of the cancer agency to run this program."

In a stroke of brilliance, Schmidt asked the subcommittee to recall the first day of testimony. The NCI director, Baker, was seated in the gallery, behind the table where the NIH director and HEW administrators were positioned. There were cards on the table giving the names of those seated there; there was none for Baker, sitting behind them. So when Baker had responded to a question from Representative Nelsen, the congressman had to ask for Baker's name. At this point in the telling, Schmidt's voice rose. "We want to get the man who's running the cancer program at this table when your committee is having hearings on cancer, not in the row behind the Secretary and Assistant Secretary, and the head of NIH and so forth. You do not want 'Dr. What's-His-Name' running the cancer program!"[17]

The subcommittee session was adjourned at three forty-five. The panel members were not invited back to the hearings.

⁓

True to his word about conducting long hearings, Rogers's committee heard testimony from thirty-one members of the House (twenty of whom favored a separate cancer agency), plus sixty-seven individuals who were not in Congress. Hundreds of pages of supporting documents and letters were submitted for the record. Rogers purposely sought more scientific witnesses from the state of Massachusetts than from any other single state, an obvious message to Senator Kennedy. His mission was laser-focused: to get *his* bill passed. Period.

The subcommittee met five more times in September and twice in early October. Before the last meeting, Mary went to see Ancher Nelsen. She had been impressed by his questioning of Senator Nelson, but she was even more impressed by his words at the end of the first day. He appeared to be a man willing to pull the sides together and able to assess what was practical in politics. For his part, Nelsen had been thinking about S. 1828's requirement that the head of the new cancer agency report directly to the president. Not only would that take the director away from his work, but it was unlikely the president would have the necessary time.

"He conceived the idea that, although Rogers would not give in and let the head of the Cancer Institute report to the President," Mary later said, "he might give in to the extent that the president have a Cancer Attack Panel. [It would be] appointed by himself and . . . would monitor what was going on in the Cancer Institute, notifying the President if there were any bureaucratic blockages." This panel would be made up of three people: Mary's favorite recipe of clinician, basic scientist, and layperson. It would also act as a liaison to Congress, thereby creating a free flow of information. Mary loved the idea and suggested he take it to ACS president Dr. Pollard and senior executive Alan Davis. They loved it as well. So on October 7, Nelsen floated his idea before the committee.

Washington Democrat Brock Adams testified first on his experience as a member of the authorizing committee for NASA's Apollo program within the Science and Astronautics Committee. Nelsen asked Brock, almost musing to himself, "In the Rogers bill you have a National Cancer Advisory Council, and they sort of sit in an overview position. And I was wondering if there is some sort of middle road in this proposition. . . . Now, if there was a little review group of two or three, appointed by the president, and with the authority of umpiring the activity, maybe we could accommodate the wishes of the so-called Senate bill. This might be a possibility, and I just toss it to you."[18]

After the hearings adjourned at four-twenty, Gorman gave Mary a full report on how Nelsen's proposal had been received. She was grateful and hopeful, but maybes weren't yeses. The cancer act had now been so dragged out that it had lost the public's attention. The Citizens Committee for the Conquest of Cancer's full-page advertisements directed at senators had been successful. So why not do it again, this time directed at Rogers's subcommittee members? Quinn was still working from his hospital bed, sending letters to as many old friends in the House as possible. When Mary called him to share her newspaper plan, he was adamant that she not do it, fearing that a repeat performance would be too heavy-handed. That dissuaded her from even consulting Benno Schmidt. Gorman, however, urged her forward, and she went through with the plan.

On Sunday, October 10, newspapers in Maine, New York, Virginia, North Carolina, Florida, Minnesota, Kentucky, Missouri, Kansas, and California ran identical ads—twenty-one in all—save for the names and addresses of the sub-committee members in each district. "This absolutely shocked the people in the House," Mary later observed. "People were calling from their districts and send-ing telegrams, and it caused quite a little commotion. They had telephone calls from people who said, 'I don't want to speak to his assistant, I want to speak to him, I'm a voter in his district!'"

Meanwhile, ignorant of Mary's plan, ACS decided to run its own full-page ads in the *New York Times*, the *Washington Post*, and the *Washington Evening Star*. "An open letter to the 435 members of the House of Representatives from the presi-dent of the American Cancer Society," the ad began.[19] It was an attempt to reach the full House, rather than just the subcommittee.

The next day, Rogers, along with subcommittee members Peter Kyros, a Democrat, and James Hastings, a Republican, was scheduled to go on a prear-ranged visit to Roswell Park Memorial Institute in Buffalo, New York. The can-cer center bordered Hastings's district, and Rogers felt the visit could be a two-fold success. First, the field trip made for great press. And second, Rogers wanted the votes of the four Republicans on the subcommittee for unanimous approval of his bill. Rogers smiled for the cameras present, but inside he was seething at the furor generated by the latest batch of advertisements—his office had received a hundred telegrams urging him to pass the Senate's version of the cancer bill.

"I don't know why anyone feels they have to go to the extent of spending large amounts of money," he told reporters, clearly taking aim at Mary. The ads' sponsors, he said, wanted to "stampede the Congress and we think it's better to look at these matters in all aspects rather than have something crammed down the throat of Congress."[20]

On October 12, the subcommittee began its four-day executive session to achieve unanimity and produce a clean bill. They would not accept the full text of S. 1828, but to get a bill passed by the entire Congress, there would have to be compromise, drawing in parts of it and the myriad other House bills. Once rewritten to everyone's satisfaction, the clean bill would receive a new number.

Their first step was to remove the reference to "major killer diseases" and institutes in H.R. 10681, on the grounds that diseases other than cancer should not be named in a cancer bill. It was something the clever Rogers had been willing to compromise on, along with the line about their directors and associates being presidential appointees. That point was left in for future bargaining. While NCI would remain in place, its director would have budget autonomy from NIH and HEW. The still-hospitalized Quinn was now making phone calls, pleading with the Republicans to hold fast and not agree to H.R. 10681 or any version of it.

When Friday rolled around, Representative Nelsen brought Rogers his fully formed idea of establishing the President's Cancer Attack Panel. That brainstorm garnered the acceptance of the last Republican holdout. The subcommittee had its clean bill, now H.R. 11302, the National Cancer Attack Act of 1971.

Paul Rogers might have fueled his House hearings with ego and stubbornness, but he was a keen politician, understanding the importance of compromise. He was joined by the bombastic Senator Nelson at a triumphant press conference that afternoon. Nelson still fumed about the ads, which he said were part of "a propaganda campaign at the grassroots level," and accused the Citizens Committee for the Conquest of Cancer of "making a political issue of an important scientific matter."[21]

No one knew more about the "important scientific matter" to which Nelson referred than Mary. Politics had nothing to do with it. Mary's motivation was her compassion for human life. According to her most recent statistics, 323,330 more Americans would die of cancer that year, while 964,000 would be in treatment for the disease. An astronomical $1.8 billion (nearly $14 billion today) would be spent for that treatment. In addition, 175,000 person-years of productivity would be lost, the equivalent of $1.2 billion in lost income (nearly $9 billion in 2023). During the testimony of the panel members, Farber had adroitly pointed out, "The Congress appropriates one and a half billion dollars a year *not* to preserve the structure of the NIH, but to preserve the health of the American people."[22] A brilliant statement if ever there was one.

Chapter 16

"The Most Sympathetic
President We've Ever Had"

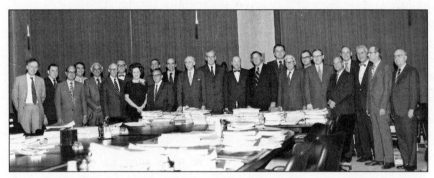

*First meeting of the National Cancer Advisory Board, March 1972. Third from the left is entertainer
Danny Thomas. Mary is the only woman. The fourth man to her left is Dr. Sidney Farber.*

B y the middle of October 1971, it would have been difficult for any
newspaper-reading American to not be at least tangentially aware of
the "war on cancer." Mary's ads, Rogers's and Nelson's indignation,
and the published letter from ACS president Pollard contributed to the onset
of a loud journalistic battle. Despite Mary's feelings and Nelson's claims that
cancer shouldn't be political, nearly every article carried the word "politics" in
either its title or its content.

The congressmen's initial belief was that the ACS letter had been connected
to Mary's Citizens Committee for the Conquest of Cancer. They accused ACS
of using donations for political purposes, a direct and potentially dangerous
violation of the organization's nonprofit status. Voicing that opinion, a *New York*

Times editorial spoke of the "high-powered advertising campaign launched by the American Cancer Society" in support of S. 1828. "The American Cancer Society," the editorial continued, "does the cause of combating cancer no favor by its campaign against the useful Rogers initiative."[1]

Step one for ACS, then, was to distance itself from the unfortunate timing of that newspaper piece. A group of concerned individuals placed the ads, an ACS spokesperson said, and "no public contributions" were used for Dr. Pollard's letter. Rogers had been quoted as claiming that "all of the other scientific community is almost unanimous in its opposition to an independent agency." Referring to the Panel of Consultants' report, the spokesperson countered, "We *are* following the recommendations of the scientific community."[2]

True to his history, Schmidt fired off a response to the *Times* editorial, arguing that the newspaper was thinking of the NCI organizational discussion as a simple "issue of right and wrong." He pointed out that seventy-nine of eighty senators, a "vast majority" of people who had spent their lives battling cancer, HEW executives, "an objective panel of consultants," and the president of the United States all stood in favor of the Senate bill. He concluded by observing that the *Times* had "an unhappy tendency" of proclaiming that those not in line with their thinking must have political motives.[3] The next day the *Times* printed another letter, this one signed by thirteen cancer doctors and researchers at Harvard. They vehemently disagreed with the claim in Pollard's letter that objection to S. 1828 came only from those *outside* the cancer world, for they themselves were part of that world.[4] The net result of all these volleys was that, once again, President Nixon's name was removed from the cancer discussion. The administration needed to regain the attention. Fortuitously, something perfect was on the back burner.

Forty miles northwest of Washington, in the town of Frederick, Maryland, was Fort Detrick, an army base that had been the headquarters of America's biological warfare research. When Nixon announced in November 1969 that he was discontinuing that project, over three hundred Frederick residents faced unemployment. So in 1970, the city council suggested using the base's labs for environmental research. But then, in January 1971, Senator Edward Muskie (another potential Nixon presidential opponent) urged that the base be used by NIH. Nixon's White House didn't reply to the suggestion.

On February 5, Maryland's two senators (both Republicans) concurred with Muskie. Fort Detrick, they said, "has laboratory facilities second to none anywhere in the world, which have been employed to handle some of the 'hot viruses' which much be investigated in an effort to find a cancer cure." The administration continued to say nothing. Nor did it make a statement when one of those senators, Charles Mathias, told a luncheon crowd that the Panel of Consultants had named Fort Detrick in their report as a potential research facility.

Mathias wrote numerous letters to HEW secretary Richardson and in March published statements from panel doctors Krim, Farber, Holland, and Clark reiterating their support for the base's conversion. The senator continued making speeches about the idea in and out of Congress. Still not a word from the White House.

Suddenly, on Friday, October 15, the Associated Press reported it had learned that Nixon was soon headed to Fort Detrick to make an announcement. Three days later, after having toured several of the buildings, the president addressed an assemblage that included Maryland's members of Congress, some Frederick residents, and a scrum of reporters.

"I am glad to see that, despite what happened to the Orioles yesterday, everybody is happy here today in Maryland." (The Orioles had lost the seventh and last game of the World Series.) The president continued, "For thousands of years, mankind has dreamed of turning swords into plowshares and spears into pruning hooks, of changing the implements of war into instruments of peace. Today we mark another chapter in the realization of that dream as we announce that one of our largest facilities for research on bacteriological warfare is being converted into a leading center for cancer research."[5]

As he ended his speech that lovely fall day, Nixon took aim. "The action of the Congress in approving my $100 million request for the cancer-cure program was an important step in the campaign against cancer. So was the vote of the Senate approving the Conquest of Cancer Act—which provides for an independently budgeted program with a director who is responsible directly to the President. I again urge the House of Representatives to act promptly on this matter so that we can get on with this important work."

Just like that, cancer fighter in chief Richard Nixon was back on page one, aiming for the big prize: a bill that would fund the end of cancer.

⁓

"In the House, they hate the Senate." Mary had honed this observation as the result of her three decades of lobbying on Capitol Hill. The two chambers' rivalry had developed nearly two hundred years earlier. They differ in more ways than they are similar (size, procedures, terms of office, constitutional responsibilities), each guarding its own power and prerogatives, generally suspicious of the other body. Although it was the only path to enact a law, rare was the occasion that both chambers readily agreed on anything. But the cancer bill danced around the edges.

No one disagreed with a national goal of curing the disease; they disagreed on how to do it. Mary saw positives in each bill. The Senate's version, sometimes referred to in the newspapers as the Lasker-Kennedy-Nixon bill—an interesting mixture if there ever was one—contained a plan she had long sought. She and Quinn had drafted a statement to that effect, to be circulated in the right places: "The Senate version contains three provisions not included currently in the House bill, namely a separate Cancer Agency within the National Institutes of Health; a newly created position as head of that agency responsible directly to the President; and sole Cancer Agency responsibility for program plans and budget."

Implied was that S. 1828 circumvented the pesky bureaucratic maze. And although that bill acknowledged that "adequate funds" needed to be spent for a cure, no specific amount was listed. The House version corrected that: $1.5 billion (nearly $11 billion today) was to be provided over a three-year period. Mary favored the House's language, having learned to never leave legislative wiggle room.

The notion that the U.S. Congress had finally recognized it should care about whether or not cancer was cured was a huge milestone, although in

Mary's opinion it had taken far too long. "You'd think that they would get a little bit more open minded," she said, "when one in four of us is going to have the disease, and one in six of us is going to die of it, under present circumstances." Given those statistics, Mary pointed out that 108 currently sitting members of the House would get cancer, as would 25 senators. It would not matter where their political allegiance fell.

Still, the volume of press coverage about cancer was nothing short of miraculous for a disease that, just a decade earlier, was barely mentioned. This was due, of course, to Mary's work. But credit wasn't forthcoming; rather, the attention brought out many who were downright anti-Lasker. Referred to with less-than-kind monikers, including "the health syndicate," "the cancer mafia," and "Mary's little lambs," those in the crusade were now in the crosshairs. And Mary was public enemy number one. Under the headline "Cancer Campaign Backfires in Controversy," Mary was described as the "millionaire head of the research foundation bearing the name of her late husband." The article acknowledged that she declined credit for the "conquest of cancer campaign," but then stated that "her footprints are clear in the complicated story of how the campaign developed." That description was a not-so-veiled suggestion that a non-scientist of significant means had somehow brainwashed her group into taking unprecedented steps to upset a status quo. Again pulling in politics, the writer revealed that Mary was among the Democratic Party's major contributors, giving $69,400 to Senator Humphrey's 1968 presidential campaign (over half a million dollars today).[6] Ironically, the press never made the same fuss about Bobst's nearly identical donation to the Nixon campaign that same year.

Mary felt most attacked by an article in the November 1971 issue of *Harper's Magazine*, "The Politics of Cancer." The author wrote, "If NIH dies because of Mary Lasker's compulsion to do something special about cancer, both science and medicine may suffer."[7] No mention was made that the NCI's annual budget had been only $550,000 when Mary Lasker began lobbying in 1946. The bill now before the House committee was recommending ten times that much. This was not a woman bent on killing NIH. "That I was going to destroy science," Mary exclaimed, speaking about the piece, "it's ludicrous!"

On Monday, November 1, two days before the House's full Committee on Interstate and Foreign Commerce began its hearings, the ever-prepared Paul Rogers sent a packet to the committee members. Signed by all the members of his subcommittee, the cover letter outlined H.R. 11302, and it was accompanied by editorials, articles, and letters that were critical of changing the relationship between NCI and NIH.[8] When the hearings began in a closed-door session, Rogers and his subcommittee felt confident in the bill's passage—first because it was a strong bill, and second, and more importantly, because many of the committee's Republicans were in their camp. A subcommittee's bill usually takes only a day for agreement. When these hearings went into a second day, Mary and the crusade took heart, suspecting that perhaps there was trouble in paradise.

On November 4, the hearings' second day, Democrat Brock Adams drew the committee's attention to a letter HEW secretary Richardson had written to each of them, urging the passage of a bill with language duplicating that of S. 1828. "Unlike H.R. 11302," Richardson wrote, "the unique organizational structure proposed by the Senate-passed bill would reflect the president's personal commitment to an intensive campaign to find a cure for cancer." In other words, the president favored S. 1828 over the House version. After the letter had been read, Adams recommended that they follow its advice. He had told a reporter earlier what he was now suggesting to his colleagues: "There would be a bitter fight with the Senate if the House does not approve the Senate version. This would lead to a real impasse."[9]

The problem with approving S. 1828 was that it would undermine the House subcommittee. In addition, it gave the Senate credit for doing a better job, something very few in the hearing room were willing to do. Adams's recommendation was voted down 24–4. The committee then took its final vote on H.R. 11302, creating the reality Mary had been fearing: 26 aye, 2 nay. (Joining Adams in the nay column was Robert Tiernan, who had come to Congress after the death of Fogarty in 1967.) More disappointing still was the fact that despite his promises to Mary—and her dependence on him—Chairman Staggers was a no-show. If he voted for the Rogers bill, his high-placed friends in the Senate would take offense. And voting for a Senate bill over its House counterpart wasn't even an option. So Staggers didn't vote at all. Adams, however, vowed to do what Staggers wouldn't: carry the fight to the House floor. "Unless there's a public outcry and some support from the president," he warned, "the House bill will pass."[10]

Mary's philosophy had always been that tomorrow would be another day. And in this case, the next day was a special one. The Waldorf Astoria, the Park Avenue site of some of the city's most luxurious events, was decked out to the nines on the evening of November 5, hosting the fifty-eighth annual ACS awards banquet. As honorary chairman of the board, Mary never missed these galas. As always, the ballroom was packed, not only to honor the awardees but also to hear from a special guest. Radiant in a floor-length pink gown, President Nixon's younger daughter, Julie Eisenhower, was introduced to a standing ovation. She had come, she said, with a message from her father: that cancer research would be "one of the greatest endeavors of the decade."[11]

After Julie retook her seat at the head table, her dinner companions were recognized for their contributions. Eppie Lederer (Ann Landers) received an award for her "extraordinary service," but the true honors went to Mary and Bobst, both receiving the very first Founders Awards. Secretary Richardson presented them after having told the throng that the president would continue to push for "the creation of a largely independent cancer agency."

"Richardson was much more friendly than I'd ever felt him to be before," Mary said of the evening. "I've never seen anyone who was so stiff and cold when I first encountered him, who later became positively friendly."

In addition to the message Nixon had sent with his daughter, he sent another that day. Putting Republicans in both the House and Senate on notice, he made it clear that he wanted a cancer bill to sign, and he wanted it before Christmas. While Rogers hadn't been directly instructed by the president, he, too, wanted the bill passed before the end of the year. The alternative might be having to start all over when Congress reconvened after the holidays, erasing the work already done. He reported H.R. 11302 to the full House on Wednesday, November 10.

Although the subcommittee and committee votes had been relatively easy,
Rogers was careful not to be too confident. Adams had mounted a good argument, and one hundred representatives had supported S. 1828 when it was first
presented. But Rogers had another problem. Congress would recess for Thanksgiving just nine days later and not return until the twenty-ninth. They would
recess for the year on December 17. If there was a floor fight, as Adams predicted,
the president might not get his Christmas wish. Suddenly the calendar, too, had
become a foe of Rogers on one side and the crusade on the other.

Making matters worse, the cancer bill was floating in a logjam of legislation awaiting House hearings in the waning days of the year. The House Rules
Committee would work H.R. 11302's hearings onto the calendar when, and if,
time could be found. There was a work-around, however, called the "suspension
of rules." It allowed a bill to be heard without waiting in line. Three stipulations
must be met: suspensions could only happen on a Monday (the congressional
day reserved for this purpose), there could only be forty minutes of debate with
no changes to the bill, and it had to pass by a two-thirds majority (as opposed to
a simple majority). Three parties had to agree to the suspension: the Speaker of
the House, the Rules Committee chair, and the presenting committee chair, in
this case, Staggers. On the afternoon of the tenth, all agreed. The House would
convene to vote on H.R. 11302 on Monday, December 15. Rogers was so close to
getting the bill, *his* bill, passed.

~

Thirty years after cardiologist John Hay had suggested it was a danger to di-
agnose high blood pressure (hypertension) because it would then have to be
treated, Mary was thrilled to present Dr. Edward Freis a 1971 Lasker Award for
doing just that. Bestowing his award at the November 12 annual luncheon was
highly significant for her. While cancer was Mary's current focus, not a day
passed that she didn't think of her parents' sudden deaths.

The awards had now become the most sought-after accolade in medicine,
referred to as the "American Nobels." "They aren't equivalent in the sense that
they don't pay as much money," Mary explained humbly. The 1971 awardees

would receive $10,000 each (the equivalent of more than $70,000 today, although the awardees now receive $250,000). The Nobel winners receive nine times that amount. "But actually," Mary went on, "we have been lucky in that our juries have selected 23 winners [who] later [received] the Nobel Prize."

The juxtaposition of the positive press surrounding the Lasker Awards and the negative press about the Laskerites couldn't have been greater. The two entities carried the same name and had the same woman—with the same passion and purpose—driving them. The dichotomy was made even clearer when President Nixon sent Dr. Freis a personal letter after the luncheon.

"My warmest congratulations to you on receiving the Albert Lasker Medical Research Award," Nixon wrote. "There can be no question that this is one of the most prestigious awards given in medical research, and it is a source of special pride to me that it was given to a member of the Federal Government medical research team."[12]

Nixon had become adept in assuming the role of America's benevolent father figure. What lay beneath was a different story.

⟜

"The best machinery in the world to lead the attack on cancer now exists in the National Institutes of Health," Dr. Philip Lee told a reporter. "Let us oil it and refuel it and shift it into high gear."[13]

As a former assistant secretary of HEW and now chancellor at the University of California, San Francisco, Lee was rabidly against taking NCI out of NIH. He had said so when testifying in the Senate hearings, and now he stood in support of Rogers's bill. Sentiments such as Lee's aggravated Mary. *If* NIH was the place to conduct cancer research, *if* there were no bureaucratic issues, *if* that institution could, indeed, achieve what the Laskerites were seeking, why had it not done so? Why did it only now decide to step up its work with the urgency that Mary had felt for most of her life?

The debate to determine the future of the "best machinery in the world" began at noon on Monday, November 15. The forty minutes of discussion were over in a flash, and the Speaker directed the clerk to call the roll. By a vote of

350 in favor and 5 opposed, H.R. 11302 was approved.[14] There were now two bills with the same general goal, the conquest of cancer—one in the House and one in the Senate. But only one bill could go to the president for signing. Both chambers would have to come together and forge a single, negotiated settlement of their differences. It would happen in a conference committee, scheduled for December 1.

During the ten days that Congress was in recess for Thanksgiving, articles about Ted Kennedy appeared in hundreds of newspapers across the country. It was neither the vital cancer legislation nor the now nearly forgotten Chappaquiddick incident that captured the attention of the press. Nestled between the last-minute grocery ads and the early Christmas shopping suggestions, the articles all pondered the same question: would Ted Kennedy be a presidential candidate in 1972? Kennedy had repeated that he was not interested, standing by the decision he had made several years earlier. And yet he was actually leading in polls of prospective candidates, further driving Nixon's paranoia. What interesting Thanksgiving dinner conversations the Kennedy and Nixon families must have had.

Mary spent the holiday as other Americans did, in the company of family and friends. There was not much more that could be done for the crusade. She could only hold out hope that Kennedy and his team, along with the supportive members of the House subcommittee, would ensure that some (if not all) of the Panel of Consultants' recommendations appeared in the final bill. The conference committee hearings would not be public. Nonetheless, Mary, Schmidt, and Clark met in D.C. the Tuesday after Thanksgiving to see their bill through to the end. Their frustration in not being able to persuade the House members to join the crusade was mirrored in the public.

Journalist Marquis Childs wrote, "A killer stalking the land defies all the barriers of law and order. It is cancer. . . . Unfortunately, the proposed program, which originated with a distinguished commission, has stirred the kind of political bureaucratic tempest that so often clouds the issues. . . . As one who has just observed a long vigil, with the killer finally triumphant, there is only one thing to say: Stop the bureaucratic quarreling and get on with it, get on with it, get on with it."[15] Childs had been on the battlefield; his wife of forty-two years had died of cancer three years earlier.

The White House, too, received emotional pleas. Beginning his "open letter to the leaders of mankind," Stanley Goldman said he was writing "this letter in a rage of frustration. Our beautiful daughter, Laurie, died of Ewing Sarcoma. . . . She was eleven years and eleven months old." He wrote of Laurie's suffering and then appealed for help. "Men who go millions of miles to photograph a rock, unleash the atom, walk on the moon, have the cure for cancer within their reach. As a father in anguish . . . , as a man in fear for your life, your loved ones as well as my own, I beg, I demand that we unite in one mighty effort to find the answer."[16]

Mary knew these men's grief. If only politics and the science would yield to their pleas.

The U.S. Constitution doesn't specify how a conference committee is to negotiate, or even who is to represent each chamber, although most often the conferees are members of the committees that reported the bills. The two versions of the cancer bill had differences as distinct as their respective architects. When the committee convened on Wednesday, December 1, Staggers, Springer, Rogers, and the other nine members of the House Public Health and Environment subcommittee sat around a table with Kennedy, Javits, and the other thirteen members of their Senate Health and Scientific Research Subcommittee, including the irascible Gaylord Nelson.

Nelson had already counseled the House conferees on probable Senate moves, and he would continue to do so to the end. For his part, Schmidt had learned that Rogers would be completely unmovable on the idea of moving NCI out of NIH. To the surprise of the House members, Kennedy and his team barely broached that subject. The bigger discussion was the makeup of the president's Cancer Attack Panel, which filled most of Wednesday's and Thursday's meetings. The senators wanted to add three more members: the directors of both NCI and NIH and the chair of the National Advisory Cancer Council (alternately called the National Cancer Advisory Council). The House members were adamantly opposed; if the panel was to be the watchdog of the work being done, putting those three on it would be akin to the fox watching the henhouse.

Rogers felt his position was strong. Not only was his entire team on board, along with Senator Nelson, but a number of other senators had let him know they preferred the House version of the bill, as well. The congressman was in the position of not really needing to negotiate much at all, and consequently sat mute most of the time, as did much of his team. Midway through the first day, Kennedy said, "Well, you act as if you're the only one who has anything to say about this. After all, the Senate passed the bill 79 to 1, *our* 79 to 1." He stormed out, and they recessed until after lunch. "I don't know what to do with them," Kennedy told Mary that evening. "I can't get anyplace with them."

More of the same continued on Thursday, with the two sides completely deadlocked. Then, in a stroke of genius, Kennedy suggested they make a weekend visit to the president to ascertain his wishes. He knew Nixon preferred S. 1828; it was Nixon's bill, after all. If the president leaned in that direction, the House conferees, and all of the House Republicans, would feel obliged to go along. But in truth, the administration (speaking through HEW) had actually taken four positions. First it opposed any legislation; then it favored only its own bill; next, members of the administration testified in the House in support of the Senate bill; and now they supported the Senate bill, with parts of the House bill attached as amendments. Translation: Nixon just wanted a bill; the House version was as good as the Senate's.

Not wanting to curtail their momentum, the House conferees rejected the idea of a visit, so Kennedy and Javits wrote letters instead. They asked for Nixon's view on their panel idea before the seventh, when the conference committee would reconvene. The president responded on the sixth, "My view is that I could work effectively with either version." What he wanted, he said, was something that "gives the person in charge of the program a high degree of independence and responsibility, so that he can cut through the red tape which so often has choked other Government programs."[17] Another deflection; it wasn't helpful, but it was sincere.

There were twenty-five days left before the end of the year, and Congress would only be in session for the next ten. Nixon was desperate for a cancer bill, *any* cancer bill. Chicago journalist Bob Wiedrich had laid it out clearly earlier in the year. "If Richard Milhous Nixon, the 37th president of the United states can achieve these two giant goals—an end to the war in Viet Nam and defeat of the ravages of cancer—then he will have carved for himself in the history of this nation a niche of more than Lincolnesque proportion."[18]

In December 1971, there were 334,600 U.S. military personnel in South Vietnam.[19] The draft was still plucking young men out of jobs and classrooms and sending them to the war, which had now expanded to Laos and Cambodia. That war would not be ending that year, and maybe not even the next year. That left only a cancer bill to elevate Nixon to "Lincolnesque proportion."

Seeing no support from the White House, to Mary's disappointment the senators accepted the House version of the Cancer Attack Panel when they met again on Tuesday. But the Senate prevailed when it came to an expanded NACC, now to be called the National Cancer Advisory Board. The House favored its original form, as described in the original 1937 Cancer Act. The new version would have eighteen members, as opposed to the current fourteen. Of those, no more than twelve could be scientists or physicians, and no more than eight would be laypeople. Nixon had liked the idea of "expanded outside influence."[20]

The Senate also prevailed in its request to remove all mention of other institutes, diseases, and directors. Rogers had anticipated this; it was an unimportant section, but its redaction gave Rogers extra negotiating points. Both bills stated that the NCI and NIH directors would be appointed by the president and report directly to him, and that the NCI budget would circumvent the NIH and HEW stopping points and go straight to the Office of Management and Budget. These ideas were revolutionary. But the Senate also wanted to exercise its power to advise and consent for each of those. "The Senate has never had advise and consent power over health matters," Staggers said bluntly, "and it will not have it now."[21] They all agreed on the creation of fifteen new cancer research centers, and the sum of $1.6 billion ($11.7 billion today) to be spent over the next five years to conquer cancer.

At the end of the third day, the conferees shook hands and emerged with the National Cancer Act of 1971. In the coming days, the committee's bill, S. 1828 (retaining its number, since that was Nixon's bill) was presented in each chamber, amid accolades and strongly supportive adjectives. Each chamber, in turn, voted to accept the bill unanimously.

Mary's summation of the war on cancer's blastoff was humbly understated: "We're beginning a new era. It's just one part of a big long road."

⬝

Thursday, December 23, was, as Mary remembered it, "a beautiful day in Washington." The unseasonably warm temperature rose to fifty degrees, and, as if smiling down in approval, the sun shone all day. Nixon had been conflicted (as he often was) about hosting a large event to officially sign the bill. It would mean sharing the stage with Kennedy. In the end, Nixon's advisors convinced him that the benefit of appearing as a compassionate cancer generalissimo would go far. The seventeen-hundred-square-foot State Dining Room was hastily set up to accommodate the more than 130 invited guests, including Mary. In the front of the room, a desk was framed by wall sconces decked with holiday greenery. And at noon, a jubilant and jovial president entered to a standing ovation.

"We are here today for the purpose of signing the Cancer Act of 1971. . . . And I hope, in the years ahead, that we may look back on this day and this action as being the most significant action taken during this administration." He spoke for another three minutes before taking a seat at the desk. "A souvenir pen will be available to everyone in the audience," Nixon said. "It's a very good pen, but the box is worth more than the pen. You get the box, too!"[22] (The president would send Mary a pen a week later "as a memento of this significant step," telling her that her presence at the signing was "particularly meaningful.")

Although Congress had officially recessed on the seventeenth and most of its members had gone home, many who had played a part in the National Cancer Act returned for the ceremony. The president invited them to gather around the desk for photos. Mary watched as Rogers, Dominick, Williams, Staggers, and Kennedy all shook hands and encircled the president. Kennedy ended up directly behind Nixon, his hand resting on the back of the president's chair. The scene might have symbolized either of two things. From one point of view, Nixon had ended up in front of the senator in the war on cancer, and was determined to remain in front throughout the rest of their political careers. From a different point of view, Kennedy had put himself in a position to watch the president's every move, his hand at the ready to pull Nixon back if need be.

At the end of the nine-minute ceremony, the president invited the attendees to enjoy coffee and a tour of the White House, decked out in its Christmas finery. As had been the case at the 1965 signing, Mary said of those in attendance, "Many of them had done their utmost to defeat the bill in one way or another. Now, they were all taking a lot of credit, and drinking coffee, and talking to each other." But she also recognized the value in the moment. "I think the White House has finally faced the fact that the NIH management is not in favor of doing anything especially dynamic. They're alerted to this. Now, what happens if Nixon's defeated? You can have a lot of trouble explaining this to another president, another set of staff and people." Allowing herself time to relish the moment, she concluded, "Nixon [might turn] out to be the most sympathetic president we've ever had."

At one-twenty that afternoon, as the last guests were leaving the White House, Nixon went to his retreat in the Executive Office Building and called special counsel Chuck Colson, who arrived twenty minutes later. The morning's triumphant president had morphed into a dark, plotting one. Nixon wanted an update on the "dirty tricks" being planned against Senator Edward Kennedy in advance of the upcoming New Hampshire primary.[23]

Chapter 17

"If You Think Research Is
Expensive, Try Disease"

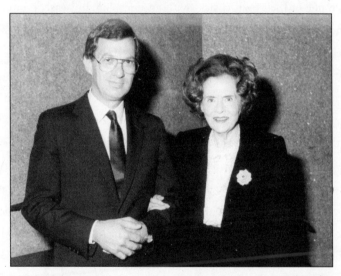

Mary with Dr. Vincent DeVita at the dedication of the Mary Woodard Lasker
Center for Health and Research Education, September 9, 1984.

A
mericans' feelings toward their most feared illness lifted somewhat
in the twenty-four months after the "war on cancer" was declared.
As with any war, however, there were casualties. Yet a projected
1.29 million Americans would be diagnosed with cancer over those two years,
and 700,000 would die.[1] Despite his valiant work to give life to the National
Cancer Act from a hospital bed, Luke Quinn died of non-Hodgkin's lymphoma
on March 12, 1972, at the age of sixty-four. Panel of Consultants member Dr.

Wendell Scott's cancer returned, and he succumbed on May 4, 1972, at sixty-six. Mary felt the loss keenly: these men's dedication to the crusade had been immeasurable.

Money didn't keep cancer at bay, either. Winthrop Rockefeller, the brother of Mary's good friend Laurance Rockefeller, was diagnosed with pancreatic cancer in September 1972. As soon as she heard, Mary called Laurance and asked, "What are they going to do for him?" "Oh, well, they're giving him some drug," Laurance replied, "but there's no hope for him."

"The Rockefellers have spent untold money to try to help Memorial [Memorial Sloan Kettering]," Mary said later, "and untold in medicine generally. But when one of their own is sick, with an unexplored disease, no matter how much money you've spent, it doesn't help you any. The information isn't there, it's hopeless." Winthrop Rockefeller would die in February 1973.

Mary would soon feel cancer's sting in her own family. Alice's husband, Al, had been diagnosed with prostate cancer in 1967. He had been treated with a drug that, just a few years earlier, had accidentally been discovered as effective against this form of the disease. It reduced Al's tumor and stabilized the cancer's growth. But the cancer came back in the spring of 1972. While Al underwent cobalt treatments, Mary persuaded the Veterans Administration to sponsor a visit by a Swedish doctor who'd had success with combination chemotherapy in prostate cancer cases. Unfortunately, the treatment came too late. Al died on September 24, 1972.

"The illness and death of Al Fordyce just reinforced me in my feeling that I have to work harder in this maze of cancer research," Mary told a friend. "I have to try to get more specific things done, as well as to be sure that we have more money." Mary may have had an unending supply of passion and purpose (accompanied by an admirable amount of energy for a seventy-three-year-old), but now both Woodard sisters had been widowed by the disease.

Neither would heart disease be tamed. And, as the number one cause of death in the country, it, too, touched Mary again. On February 11, 1972, three doctors worked on a sixty-two-year-old woman named Diana who had just suffered a crushing heart attack. Diana had come to Houston's Methodist Hospital, where Michael DeBakey was working. She had a history of heart attacks, having had one just a few weeks earlier. The doctors' work was in vain; Diana died. She was Dr. DeBakey's wife of thirty-five years.

Several years earlier, and at Mary's insistence, Lyndon Johnson had become a patient of DeBakey's. LBJ had gained weight and returned to smoking after leaving the presidency. The result was heart attacks in 1970 and 1972. On January 22, 1973, having lost weight but still smoking, Johnson suffered his final heart attack at his Texas ranch at the age of sixty-four. Mary was saddened by the death of her friend, only to feel that grief again two months later. Dr. Sidney Farber's colorectal cancer was still a secret; not even Mary knew. But while he survived this cancer, his heart betrayed him. On March 30, 1973, Farber was found dead in his Boston lab, having suffered a fatal heart attack.

Some years earlier, when an interviewer had asked why Mary was so adamant about medical research, she had replied, "I am opposed to heart disease and cancer the way one is opposed to sin." If only that fierceness could have tamed the diseases; if only Nixon's enthusiasm about "his" National Cancer Act had been sincere.

After resoundingly beating George McGovern in the 1972 election, Nixon no longer needed to be seen as slayer-in-chief of the scourge. Consequently, cancer was no longer politically attractive—or important—and the president's actions made that abundantly clear. His administration's first program update, as required by the Cancer Act, appeared more than two hundred days late. And his budget office cut the fiscal 1974 NCI budget by $140 million, against strong opposition from Congress, NIH, and his own President's Cancer Panel (previously called the Cancer Attack Panel).

Then, in a January 31, 1973, news conference, Nixon went a step further. "The constitutional right for the President of the United States to impound funds—and that is not to spend money, when the spending of money would mean either increasing prices or increasing taxes for all the people—that right is absolutely clear."[2] He was correct: it is a constitutional right, but not if it's used to frustrate the will of Congress, which was precisely what was happening. The health community was enraged, no one more so than Mary.

"The truth is that Congress has the right to appropriate funds," she fumed. "And it's unconstitutional for him to impound large amounts." Now it was her turn to be correct; the constitution places a percentage cap on how much can be frozen. "He gave no money at all to regional medical centers, wiped out money," she continued. "He was legislating by impoundment. It is unheard of."

Of the funds Nixon impounded, $58,859,000 were for cancer research. Mary now realized her misplaced belief in his sincerity, saying angrily, "A friend of mine wrote me and said, 'What's going on in your country? It sounds like a combination of a banana republic and the Third Reich.'" Some citizens in the health community were so enraged, including Gorman, they took the unprecedented step of suing the administration.

Nixon, however, had bigger problems. Nearly a year earlier, his "dirty tricks" team had broken into the Democratic National Committee headquarters in the Watergate Complex and bugged several telephones. A few weeks later, one of the listening devices needed repair, so the team returned. This time they were caught, and gradually they (and others) began to talk. Soon Mary and the rest of the nation were swept up in the cloak-and-dagger drama that was unfolding. Newspaper stories overflowed with words like "scandal," "cover-up," and "perjury."

But Mary and those in the cancer world read other stories in those same papers that used words they couldn't help but be enthusiastic about: "immunotherapy," "virology," and "chemotherapy." Each, she said, "should be pursued energetically." And that was precisely what was happening. That research had begun even before the National Cancer Act was working its way through Congress. Dr. Robert Good had been intrigued with the body's ability to protect itself via the immune system. Like with any army, the soldiers of the immune system detect and then respond to invaders, everything from viruses to parasitic worms, from a wood splinter to cancer. Good began studying bone marrow, home base for the production of infection-fighting blood cells. But when that system goes awry—as in the case of leukemias, in which the marrow produces too many cells that are abnormal and don't function properly—humans die. The first bone marrow transplant was done in 1956, in which recipient and donor were identical twins. Good expanded the possibilities by saving the life of a child in 1968 with the first bone marrow transplant from a relative. He received a 1970 Lasker Award for the achievement, and a year later was named an original member of the President's Cancer Panel (along with Schmidt and Clark). By that time, Dr. Good was asking a provocative question: Could a strengthened immune system (immunotherapy) fend off cancer? Based on what she had read, Mary was an ardent supporter of that theory.

The companion research to that of immunology was virology. Scientists had begun searching for cancer viruses in the 1950s, believing they could then create a magic bullet, as had been done with polio. In fact, leading the charge in that hypothesis (from his Fort Detrick lab) was Dr. Albert Sabin, who had developed the oral polio vaccine in the early 1960s. Elsewhere, it had just been discovered that cervical cancer cells gave off a mystery chemical akin to herpes type 2, the virus that causes cold sores. As Good told an interviewer in 1973, "If we can identify a virus, we're awfully good at preventing disease . . . in a reasonably innocuous way."[3] But therein lay the problem. Cancer viruses in animals, primarily mice and monkeys, had been isolated, but their human counterpart had, as yet, eluded discovery. Still, these were the out-of-the-box ideas that made Mary's heart race.

In chemotherapy, too, tremendous strides were being made. Dr. Emil Freireich had arrived at NCI in 1955, where he met another oncologist with an oddly similar name, Dr. Emil Frei III. Ten years later, the two doctors moved to M. D. Anderson as a team, charged with creating a chemotherapy program. Cancer cells, Freireich and Frei rationalized, sometimes became resistant to a single drug. This had been Farber's motivation for giving children with leukemia several drugs, individually but in succession. Now, the two researchers wondered what might happen if they gave a cocktail of drugs simultaneously. Their experimentation was long and filled with contention, as medical counterparts across the country warned that their poisonous stew would kill patients. But they carried on and found success, inducing long-term remissions for lymphoma and acute leukemia. They, too, won a Lasker Award.

"I think the next five years will change the picture very much," Mary enthused at the time. "But the next ten years will certainly provide a profound change, if we continue to get the money. . . . I really think there's no need to talk about 20 or 30 years for the conquest of cancer. I think it can be done in this decade."

On March 18, 1974, the director of the National Cancer Institute and the National Cancer Program (created by the Cancer Act), Dr. Frank Rauscher, sent a letter to 29 Beekman Place. It began, "Dear Mary: Thank you for your letter of January 7, 1974. You are absolutely correct, of course, when you say that we can't go on asking for more money from the president and the Congress unless we demonstrate progress in the clinical area."[4] Rauscher went on for seven pages, explaining the program's new approach to solid tumors and promising to send her a list of the combination chemotherapy trials underway.

That report brought the kind of news Mary had been waiting for. As an example, the prognosis in breast cancer patients whose disease had spread to their lymph nodes was a 43 percent chance of recurrence within eighteen months. After surgery, high doses of drugs were then administered to attempt to stop the progression. But new trials were showing that giving combination chemotherapy immediately upon diagnosis reduced reoccurrence by 95 percent over a two-and-a-half-year period. Perhaps Mary's "simple pill" against cancer was out there; it just had to be discovered. Her hopes rose two months later when she met Dr. Jordan Gutterman.

Gutterman had become interested in blood diseases in medical school, ultimately focusing on hematology. He completed his residency at the height of the Vietnam War and was required to fulfill a two-year military assignment, for which he was sent to Brooke Army Hospital in San Antonio, Texas. One day, a group of doctors from Houston's M. D. Anderson Cancer Center arrived to make a presentation. Among these specialists in the new field of oncology was Dr. Emil Freireich. Gutterman instantly revered him: "He was brilliant, bold, and courageous. And he broke all the rules in terms of doing clinical things that people never heard of before."[5]

As soon as his military stint was completed, Gutterman accepted an appointment at M. D. Anderson as an assistant professor, which allowed him to also work on hematology research with Freireich. In May 1974, Dr. Lee Clark (M. D. Anderson's president) called Gutterman to tell him that Mary Lasker was coming for a visit. Gutterman knew the Lasker name from Freireich's 1972 award. Clark said he was putting together a panel of eight researchers to share their current work with Mary, and wanted Gutterman to be a part of it.

Gutterman had already determined he wanted to do something new and different in the cancer world. He had become intrigued with the immune system a year earlier. As he explained in his presentation to Mary, "Chemotherapy is great as far as what it has accomplished, but there is much to be done." Chemo cured some forms of the disease, the doctor explained, but there were others, like pancreatic cancer, that it didn't touch. However, there was a possibility of using new technology enlisting the body's own proteins to fight disease. Everything from common colds to chicken pox and (hopefully) cancer might be conquered.

Mary liked what she heard from this young doctor. She identified with people whose energy, passion, and enthusiasm matched hers. Gutterman certainly had those and more. After all the others had spoken that day, Mary approached him. "I'm really interested in your ideas of immunotherapy," she said. "Do you ever get to New York City?" She invited him to lunch at Beekman Place. As it happened, Gutterman had been invited to give two lectures in the city, three weeks apart, with the first occurring relatively soon. Mary attended both of his presentations.[6]

The prodigious cancer file that sat on her desk overflowed with articles about immunotherapy, and about one of the proteins Gutterman spoke of in particular: interferon. Occurring naturally in the blood, the substance was discovered by two researchers in London in 1957. They noticed that when patients had one viral illness, they practically never came down with a second virus at the same time. The body apparently stimulated the production of cells that interfered with further assaults, thus the name.

Since that discovery, Finnish virologist Kari Cantell had devoted all his time to the creation and study of interferon. Swedish oncologist Hans Strander had worked with Cantell and in 1972 used interferon to successfully treat children with a rare and deadly form of bone cancer. Although they didn't understand exactly how it worked, interferon appeared to block the uncontrolled division of cancer cells. Then, like a biological Paul Revere, interferon put out a call to the body's own immune system to kill the cancer cells.[7]

But interferon was hard to come by. It was species-specific, and so it could only be produced from human blood for human benefit. And it couldn't be mass-produced but had to be painstakingly harvested in a multistep process. First, a centrifuge separated blood into its three parts: the heavy red cells at the bottom, the lighter plasma on the top, and a thin layer of white cells, the color of watered-down apple cider, in between. The white cells were then infected with a virus to activate interferon production, and that concoction was spun again, resulting in impure interferon. Even after more steps, only .014 ounces of somewhat impure interferon could be produced from 90,000 pints of blood. In 1974, the entire world supply wouldn't even fill a milk bottle.

Price, too, was a problem. One-millionth of an ounce of pure interferon cost $1,500 to produce, far more expensive per ounce than gold. Nonetheless, Strander's work was exciting, and news of it had reached Mary and Gutterman individually before they even met. Each in their own way had sought a magic bullet against the world's most terrifying and psychologically daunting disease. Could this be it? If so, it was a highly unknown form of magic.

On May 9, 1974 (at nearly the same time Mary visited M. D. Anderson), there wasn't a single newspaper article about interferon. But there were thousands of newspapers carrying stories about another topic new to Americans' ears: impeachment. The Watergate break-in nearly two years before, helped along by the revelation that the president had taped conversations in both the White House and his off-site office, had led to indictments of members of President Nixon's innermost circle. The House Judiciary Committee had voted to begin impeachment hearings.

Despite Nixon proclaiming that he wasn't a crook, key Republican senators met with the president to inform him that there were enough votes to convict him. On August 8, 1974, Richard Nixon became the first American president to resign his office. Cancer still wasn't cured, as he had promised to do thirty-two months earlier. But it now appeared that his claim when signing the National Cancer Act that the act was "the most significant action taken during this administration" might well be true.

～

Despite the breadth of Mary's art collection, she rarely sent pieces out on loan. She felt certain she'd miss them, as if they were living beings in her home. The few times she did loan them, it was always when she was out of town. One of her favorite collections was of paintings and sketches by Léonard Tsuguharu Foujita. The Japanese-born artist had lived in France most of his life, his work reflecting that influence. Many of his pieces were inspired by Renoir, another of Mary's favorites. She gave Lady Bird Johnson one of her Foujitas as a gift. "If you ever need money, sell the Foujita to the Japanese," Mary had advised her friend; "[they] are in the habit of paying outrageous prices for his paintings."[8] In the summer of 1977, she decided to take her own advice.

Interferon research was moving at a crawl. For nearly three years, she and Gutterman had made many attempts to get NCI to put funds into the project. The answer was always the same, harking back to the proverbial chicken-and-egg issue: there wasn't enough data, so they weren't interested in further investigation, and because interferon was rare and expensive, limiting in-depth clinical trials, there wouldn't be more data to interest NCI to take it further. Around and around they went until Mary was beside herself with frustration.

"A Japanese dealer offered me four hundred thousand dollars for eight Foujitas," Mary explained (nearly $2 million today). "I thought this was quite a lot of money. I actually didn't need the Foujitas, and I would love to have that money to do this [fund interferon research]." Keeping one painting and one drawing, she took the money and telephoned Gutterman. "If I give you a million dollars, will you go to Sweden and Finland to see if you can buy interferon and start clinical trials? We've got to get going."

Mary had never been one to go halfway on anything, and the timing of her call was significant. Jane McDonough, Mary's secretary and friend for nearly thirty years, had had breast cancer two years earlier. Despite a double mastectomy, her cancer came back. And, as was the case when anyone she cared about was ill, Mary went to all extremes to help. But Jane's cancer had spread too far for interferon to help. She would die on March 10, 1980.

Mary persevered nevertheless, and the shopping expedition was launched two months later. Gutterman and Deeda Blair went to Stockholm to meet with Strander and Cantell. There, with Mary's investment, they purchased a huge share of the world's supply of interferon. It arrived at M. D. Anderson in early February 1978 and Gutterman went immediately to work, administering it to thirty-eight patients, including seventeen women with advanced breast cancer. He saw immediate—perhaps magical—responses.

Several years earlier, as director of NCI, Dr. Frank Rauscher, too, had sent a team to Sweden to look at Strander's bone cancer research. The institute then co-sponsored a 1975 interferon conference, which Mary, Deeda Blair, and Gutterman attended. But Rauscher just couldn't believe the results and dragged his feet. Now, in 1978, he was an ACS senior vice president and chief of research. Mary had encouraged Gutterman to report his findings to ACS. His results, along with new data from Strander and a report of increased production from Cantell, persuaded Rauscher that interferon was the real deal. And when he learned that it was Mary who had spent her own money for the purchase of the material, he was shocked into action.

"The Cancer Society has just notified me that they are going to put two million dollars into the purchase of interferon," Mary reported excitedly. "I've already spent two hundred and sixty thousand dollars, and I've promised to spend about another five hundred and fifty. Now, it may be that they will pay for the remaining and I won't have to spend that five hundred and fifty!"

Rauscher was cautiously optimistic. "The only way to find out if interferon is any good, is to buy the material and get the research started."[9] That statement was the result of Mary's insistence that ACS fund clinical trials. She also cleverly recommended that Rauscher and Gutterman be in charge of the project. They all realized the only way to get credibility for their work was to spread the trials across multiple institutes, treating multiple types of cancer: breast, lymphoma, melanoma, multiple myeloma.

Pharmaceutical companies were also watching closely, of course. Familiar names of the time like Merck, Biogen, Schering, Hoffman-LaRoche, and others began developing techniques for mass production of interferon. As the train began gathering momentum, academia got involved as well. The Massachusetts Institute of Technology began working on a technique to bring interferon's cost down. At a price tag of $150 a day per patient, up to $30,000 for a full course of treatment ($540 and $108,000 in today's money), cost would be a crucial component. Biotechnology was about to become a household word.

⁓

Ronald Reagan became president on January 20, 1981. He was an outsider, although he had governed the state of California from 1967 to 1975. His presidential campaign promises of less government and lower taxes translated almost immediately into NIH budget cuts, although throughout his presidency he insisted he supported biomedical research. Mary complained bitterly that anything costing more money was being ignored by the administration.

Given her winter weeks spent in Palm Springs with Albert, now replaced by three months in a rented Beverly Hills villa, she certainly moved in the Reagans' circle. "I've been friendly with Mrs. Reagan," Mary said matter-of-factly. However, she wasn't convinced that would make any difference in the president's policies. "They have four friends that I know that have cancer. If those people die, it might come over them that something should have been done to prevent it." One of those friends was Alfred Bloomingdale—heir to the Bloomingdale department store fortune—who would indeed die of throat cancer at the age of sixty-six. But his death did nothing to wake the Reagan administration up to the need for more disease research.

While her proverbial plate always overflowed with health projects, Mary's summer pilgrimages to Europe remained firmly on her calendar. And 1981 was no different. She spent her usual month on the Riviera, after which she and

Deeda Blair went to Venice and then Paris. In early October—despite Congress considering an important funding bill—they made a last stop at the home of a London friend. Mary became increasingly fatigued, and one night she went to bed early with a book. Her maid found her unconscious on her bathroom floor the next morning. An ambulance was summoned: Mary had suffered a stroke.[10]

Word spread quickly, and a tsunami of concern swelled. Like others, Gutterman worried he might never see her again, until he got a phone call from a British nurse. Mary came on the phone, and before any pleasantries she asked weakly, "How much money did we get from the resolution? Jordan, we've got to push to get as much money as we can when I get back."[11] She was home on the first of November, and although those close to her tried to keep her quiet, she was determined to attend the Lasker Awards a few weeks later. She made a dramatic entrance in a wheelchair, wearing her mink coat and a big smile.[12] The world of medical research exhaled a collective sigh of relief.

Mary and Mathilde Krim had become close friends. It wasn't surprising; Mathilde's husband, Arthur, had known the Laskers for years. A fellow Democrat and a movie studio head who was involved in many of the same Jewish organizations as Albert, they had much in common. Albert never knew Mathilde Galland, the beautiful Italian doctor Arthur married in 1958, but Mary liked her instantly. In addition to becoming an important part of Mary's crusade, Krim had been just as interested in researching interferon as Dr. Gutterman had.

Through her interferon laboratory at Sloan Kettering Cancer Center, Mathilde met fellow researcher Dr. Joseph Sonnabend, who was also working on the virus-killer's mysteries. Sonnabend eventually went into private practice, and one day in the spring of 1982, he shared with Krim that he was caring for an increasing number of Kaposi's sarcoma patients. The rare and deadly skin cancer quickly invaded organs and was complicated by catastrophically compromised immune systems, choking out patients' lives. By September, the bizarre condition had a name: acquired immunodeficiency syndrome, or AIDS.[13]

Along with her work in cancer, Krim learned all she could about AIDS. One of its most disturbing elements was the public's indifference to it. AIDS seemed to strike primarily sexually active gay men. If mental illness and cancer had been taboo to mention in public, talking about homosexuality took taboo to a new level. Only three stories about AIDS were published in the *New York Times* in 1981, all buried on the inside pages. So were the three published in 1982. (The president wouldn't utter the word in a major speech until 1987, at which time the disease had already struck 36,058 Americans, killing 20,849 of them.)

Krim watched her friend Sonnabend struggling to both care for patients (many of whom he treated at no cost) and try to find answers about the terrifying disease, all the while going further into debt. She had also watched Mary work over the decades, and attended many Lasker Award luncheons. Now she was driven to act. Krim presented Sonnabend with a proposal using the Lasker Foundation as a guide. With Arthur's encouragement, she wanted to begin a private research campaign against AIDS, called the American Medical Foundation (AMF). Sonnabend would direct it, while juggling his patients and research without the financial strain. Krim would be chair of the foundation, make sure it was funded and, more importantly, make it visible in the nonprofit world.

Mathilde had sought Mary's help in putting AMF together; she was also the first person Mathilde invited to join the board of directors. Mary gratefully accepted, as did others she knew from the medical research world.[14] Her humility would have undoubtedly prevented her from realizing something prophetic in the June 1983 birth of AMF. Not only was the Lasker Foundation continuing to support important researchers, but its successful template would now be used in the struggle to save more lives from this new killer.

At first glance, interferon seemed to be the perfect treatment agent for AIDS. But Sonnabend soon found that it wasn't. It actually made the disease worse, as patients developed fevers and an inability to produce white blood cells, the body's fighting army. Gutterman, too, was finding issues with interferon. Its side effects were similar to those of a viral infection, which some patients couldn't tolerate. It also seemed to be only randomly successful in sending cancer into remission, finding greatest success against hairy cell leukemia.

By this time, Gutterman was serving on the Lasker Award jury. He, DeBakey, and other close friends and advisors had gathered to discuss the blizzard of applications they'd soon receive. Mary was typically at her Beverly Hills villa and the members of the jury were happy to gather in the ritzy, star-studded city. She never traveled to California alone; her beautiful white siamese cat, Marshmallow, had become a constant companion. When Gutterman, Mary's nephew, Jim, Deeda Blair, and several others arrived for their March 1983 meeting, the dining room table was already set with elegant china, crystal, and silver.

They took their places around the table, and lunch was served. Just at that moment, Marshmallow jumped onto the table, sauntered to the middle, and began grooming himself. Mary was horrified. "Marshmallow! Get down!" she commanded. The cat paused and fixed his large blue eyes on hers of the same color. A momentary battle of wills ensued, and then he went back to his grooming. "You're just like those guys down at the NIH," Mary fumed. "They do just exactly what they want, too!"[15]

A few days later, Terry Lierman arrived at his office at a D.C. venture capital firm and found a one-way ticket to Los Angeles. No letter, no return voucher. His secretary was as stymied as he was. By this time, Lierman was practically an old-timer in the capital. He had come to Washington from Wisconsin as a conscientious objector in 1971, promising God that if he didn't get thrown in jail, he'd devote his life to public service. And what an amazing life it became. Through mentors, he landed administrative jobs at NIH and then became an intern for the Senate Labor, Health and Human Services Subcommittee under Warren Magnuson, Mary's longtime friend. When the senator was elevated to the full appropriations committee, he took Lierman with him as a staffer.

Lierman was sitting at his desk outside Magnuson's office one day in 1975 when, as he explained, "a tornado blew in. Dressed elegantly and in charge of the world, I met Mary Lasker." It was love at first sight. Magnuson lost his 1980 reelection bid, so Lierman moved on to a venture capital career. But Mary never forgot him. It was she who had sent the ticket beckoning him to California. And she called the next day to confirm his arrival. "Come see me in Beverly Hills for a few days. I want to talk to you about politics and Washington."[16]

So Lierman went. After a discussion on health issues, Mary began ticking off a list of what needed to get done. "I'd like to hire you to be my eyes and ears in D.C.," she explained. At seventy, Gorman was ready to retire; this would be a passing of the baton. Lierman protested that he knew nothing about politics. "Think about it," Mary told him, "and tell me how much you want." Lierman went home and conjured up what he thought would be the most outrageous figure for someone with his lack of experience. "I'll need $25,000 a year," he told her. Mary never blinked and gave him his marching orders.

It turned out he was, indeed, intellectually equipped to do what Mary needed done in Washington. But their relationship was also familial. He spent time every month with her at her new summer home in Greenwich, Connecticut, twelve thousand stunning square feet set on five acres that sloped down to Greenwich Bay. He visited her in New York City, too, at her new dramatic, almost baronial residence in a building at UN Plaza that boasted a who's who of business titans, politicians, and celebrities. Mary had combined two apartments into a grand, modern one perched high above the East River and just a couple of blocks from Beekman Place.

No matter where they conducted business, Lierman learned from her, loving his new career. The year after his initial trip to Beverly Hills, he left venture capital behind and created Capitol Associates, a health policy firm. He collected other medicine-related clients (with Mary's blessing, of course). And he got to know her friends, too, including Dr. Robert Gallo. "He was almost laughed out of science for believing that viruses caused cancer," Lierman remembered.[17] Gallo proved them wrong, winning a Lasker Award for precisely that, his first of two.

Lierman began to understand what motivated this now eighty-five-year-old woman. "She just really cared," he explained. "She wasn't self-promoting; she was selfless. She couldn't be pigeonholed, and she didn't just want to treat illness and disability. Her purpose in life was clear: to promote the prevention and cure for any disease." So how was it, then, that this woman who had given so much had received nothing in return? Lierman was determined to change the status quo.

During his days on the NIH campus, Lierman's office window overlooked a convent that had been grandfathered in when the government acquired the real estate. Lierman had watched the cloistered Sisters of the Visitation walk through their gardens and in and out of their beautiful eighty-year-old convent, known as the Cloisters. Now the two-story redbrick building was vacant, and Lierman thought Mary's name should be on the building. Lierman went to Speaker of the House Tip O'Neill (another old friend of Mary's) to expedite a bill approving the building's new use. On May 3, 1984, O'Neill made a statement on the House floor: "Mary Lasker is a giver, not just of what she has, but of herself. . . . Through her tireless efforts and generous determination, she has given spirit and guts to the battle against cancer and other diseases. . . . The Mary Woodard Lasker Center for Health Research and Education will be a fitting tribute to this wonderful person."[18] Lierman had come up with the building's name based on Mary's belief that research was fine, but health education would prevent disease.

He was excited to tell Mary about his plan. Mary, however, became angry, one of the few times he ever saw her angry. She didn't feel she deserved any credit for her efforts; it was Congress that deserved the credit.

And then the wheels almost came off the whole thing.

The bill had passed the House and went on to the Senate, where it also passed. But Lierman soon learned that the Howard Hughes Institute was in the process of placing investigators in host research facilities for collaboration. NIH director Dr. James Wyngaarden had nearly completed a deal for them to work out of the Cloisters. Lierman called Wyngaarden's office and was told he was in a meeting. He insisted on talking to Wyngaarden immediately, who left the meeting to come to the phone. Lierman explained their problem. "We can find another building for you," Wyngaarden said.

"No, we can't. I want *that* building." For Lierman, the building had character and pizzazz, just like Mary.

"I don't know if we can do that."

Lierman explained, "Well in about an hour, there's going to be a bill passed by the full Congress for that building to be dedicated to Mary. So whatever deal you've made, unmake it."[19]

⁓

The sun shone brightly in Bethesda, Maryland, on Sunday, September 9, 1984. Cars choked the road around the Cloisters as a crowd of several hundred made their way to their seats. Members of Congress, doctors, a few celebrities, and many friends were all there. So were Alice Fordyce and her son, Jim, along with his wife and sons. When the woman who hated making speeches—dressed in royal blue, bouffant hair and signature jewelry in place—approached the microphone, it was to a standing ovation.

"The fruits of our labors throughout the years," she told the audience, "will alleviate pain where there is suffering; provide the freedom to live in health, so that we can fulfill our promise and quest in the pursuit of happiness; and provide hope where none existed before. . . . Our leaders must realize the funding for medical research saves lives and eliminates suffering. It also saves over $13 in our economy for every $1 invested. We must all come to the immediate conclusion that if you think research is expensive, try disease!

"Thank you for coming to this dedication. Now, we must all go and continue our work."[20]

Epilogue

"Because I Value Human Life"

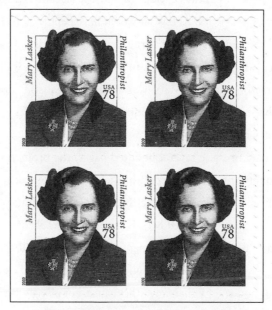

The U.S. Postal Service issued a 78-cent Mary Lasker stamp on May 15, 2009.

Mary Lasker's remarkable life ended on February 21, 1994. From nearly the beginning of her ninety-four years she had been ahead of her time, with passion and resolve that might have been perceived as "unfeminine" and "unbefitting" of her station. Dr. Vincent DeVita's memory of their first meeting paints a terrific picture of Mary's complicated persona. "With brown hair coiffed in a perfect bouffant, a mink coat slung carelessly over a chair, and perfectly applied makeup, Mary had the appearance of a lightweight socialite with too much time on her hands. Except that even when she was eyeing herself in her compact mirror, which she did often, she was listening."[1] And you can bet her mind was working.

Once called the "fairy godmother of medical research," she broke dozens of glass ceilings and was recognized in countless ways, from honorary university degrees to local and national accolades and even a postage stamp issued in 2009. The stamp's caption of "philanthropist" is laughable for those who understand the scope of her accomplishments.

As a biographer, I'm always curious to know what motivates someone to act as altruistically as Mary did. And what would have happened to NIH and medical research if she hadn't acted? It's true that the mysteries of cancer were not understood then, and they still are not. In fact, at the time the war on cancer was unfolding, detractors claimed Mary was raising unrealistic expectations, and later sneered that her influence had diminished as a result. To which I respond (perhaps a bit defensively), so what?

As you've read in these several hundred pages, she brought together Democrats and Republicans, rich and poor, in the name of combating diseases that affect us all. Jonas Salk accurately described her as "a matchmaker between science and society." Mary described herself simply in the February 10, 1958, issue of *Life* magazine: "Because I value human life, I hope *Life* will continue to alert people to what someone has called the gift of life." The cure of cancer consumed more of her time and energy than any other cause, but along with bringing it out of the shadows, she did the same with birth control, mental health, preventative heart care, and AIDS.

In its seventy-eight years, the Lasker Foundation has awarded millions of dollars, with award amounts growing from the original $1,000 to the present $250,000. It has brought public awareness to more than four hundred researchers and their work, ninety-five of whom have gone on to become Nobel laureates. Equally important, it continues to strive toward Mary and Albert's original 1942 mission: "to promote health through education and research." It's difficult to discern whether the foundation inspired Mary's successful work in lobbying, or the lobbying inspired the growth of the foundation. Either way, in her words, "we all share in the eventual glory."

Mary created the concepts of citizen lobbyists and expert witnesses, both of which transformed the way congressional testimony is heard. Her National Cancer Act also caused Congress to consider a different way of legislating and funding research. She embedded the tradition of the lay public being involved in NIH advisory boards—a role she often filled herself—along with other bodies previously closed to mere citizens. Her insistence that interferon be considered as "the simple pill," right down to putting her money where her mouth was, ignited biomedical research. That, in turn, has led to cloning and other scientific miracles she never could have conceived of when Albert told her that federal financial support would be her ticket to success.

As if those accomplishments weren't enough, the flowers that still bloom on Park Avenue, Roosevelt Island, in front of the United Nations Plaza, and elsewhere in New York are physical reminders of the woman who said they were "just little things to keep me from being depressed until a cure is found for diseases." The nation's capital is equally blessed with reminders of her generosity.

I can't help but wonder what Mary might be tuned into today. Her friend Dr. Jordan Gutterman says the plague of the future isn't infections but diseases of the brain. He thinks they would top her list. He told me, "Neurodegenerative diseases, depression, psychological diseases—they need a Mary Lasker."[2] As a cancer survivor myself, I would also selfishly lobby her to go back to her roots and continue her moon shot to end cancer. I would ask her to encourage every scientist to follow every lead and harass every legislator to fund their research.

Mary commented in 1967, "I would love to have someone write about me when I have finally given up trying to get things done. My life might even make quite a good musical." I don't have musical skills, but I certainly hope she would approve of my telling of her story. And although I never met her, I did have a role model I often thought about in writing this book. My Aunt Ethel and I were incredibly close. Even though I was an adult when my mother died, she stepped into that role when I needed a mother figure. While she didn't have the wealth

Mary did, she was more than comfortable. And as a well-respected woman of society, she broke more than her share of glass ceilings. Aunt Ethel was fifteen years younger than Mary, but I suspect they would have been good friends.

In my office, next to my favorite picture of Aunt Ethel, I have an iconic photo of a smiling Mary, seated in her white living room, surrounded by white lilies. It has been my inspiration over the nearly two years I worked on her biography. I now hope her story will be an inspiration to all researchers who dare to dream, and to all citizens who dare to challenge the status quo.

Acknowledgments

The expression "it takes a village" is never more appropriate than when writing a book. There were many who lent me a helping hand, and they are more than deserving of recognition.

The archivists at the National Archives in Washington, D.C., provided great insight into all of the congressional materials, while Library of Congress librarians chased down many newspaper and magazine articles. On the NIH campus, a team from the National Library of Medicine, the Office of History, and the Mary Lasker Center for Health Research and Education provided a wealth of historical treasure in the form of documents and photos.

Columbia University's Oral History Department dug up missing transcript pages nearly as soon as I requested them. Meanwhile, Lasker Foundation president Claire Pomeroy and senior program director David Keegan patiently answered my questions, sent lists of awardees, and provided a number of the book's photos. Melissa Lampe of the Watertown Historical Society gave me unrestricted access to Mary's family photos, her mother's memoir, and other elements crucial to this book.

The few remaining who knew Mary were likewise patient with my questions and quest for details. Whether on the phone, via Zoom, or in person, Chris Brody, Dr. Marshall Fordyce, Jim Fordyce, Dr. Jordan Gutterman, Dr. Robert Gallo, and Terry Lierman spoke eloquently and adoringly about Mary.

Two friends, Cindy Schmidt and the late Diedre Alexander, not only read chapters but encouraged me throughout the process. And when insecurity struck, they pulled out that encouraging line from *The Help*: "You is kind, you is smart, you is important."

This is the first book that Dani Segelbaum (my agent), Daniela Rapp (my editor), and I have worked on together. I think these ladies are nearly as much in love with Mary as I am. Their enthusiasm in seeing this book through to publication has been a treasure.

And finally, I am blessed with a terrific family. My children and grandchildren have watched me put together this story. I hope, when they read it, they'll understand why I've been so awestruck by Mary. Lastly, to my wonderful husband, David: you are my rock, my cheerleader, and my love.

Thank you all from the bottom of my heart.

Notes

Prologue

1. "Lasker, Pioneer in Advertising, Dies of Cancer," *Allentown* (PA) *Morning Call,* May 30, 1952, Newspapers.com.
2. "Cancer Deaths," *Mexico* (MO) *Weekly Ledger,* Dec. 11, 1952, Newspapers.com.

Chapter 1: "New York Was the Place!"

1. "Bowery Bank Lends $700,000 for New Madison Ave. Flat," *New York Tribune,* July 23, 1920, Newspapers.com.
2. "New Allerton Club Designed for Women," *New York Herald,* Nov. 5, 1922, Newspapers.com.
3. Paulina Bren, *The Barbizon: The Hotel That Set Women Free* (New York: Simon and Schuster, 2021).
4. "Grace Drake Is Director Women's Club-Hotel," *Buffalo Courier,* Sept. 30, 1923, Newspapers.com.
5. "Zuloaga Personally Conducted," *Brooklyn Daily Eagle,* Jan. 4, 1925, Newspapers.com.
6. Barbara A. Dreyer, "Adolf Meyer and Mental Hygiene: An Ideal for Public Health," *American Journal of Public Health* 66, no. 10 (Oct. 1976): 998.
7. "Women Painters Active in Circulating-Picture Plan," *Brooklyn Times Union,* Aug. 30, 1931, Newspapers.com.

Chapter 2: "That Man Is Making a Great Mistake"

1. John Gunther, *Taken at the Flood: The Story of Albert D. Lasker* (New York: Harper and Brothers, 1960), 35–37.
2. Gunther, *Taken at the Flood,* 39.
3. Gunther, *Taken at the Flood,* 54.
4. Gunther, *Taken at the Flood,* 14.
5. Jeffrey L. Cruikshank and Arthur W. Schultz, *The Man Who Sold America: The Amazing (but True!) Story of Albert D. Lasker and the Creation of the Advertising Century* (Boston: Harvard Business Review Press, 2010), 263–264.
6. Gunther, *Taken at the Flood,* 55.
7. Antoinette Donnelly, "Restyling Yourself," *New York Daily News,* Apr. 7, 1935, Newspapers.com.
8. Nancy Randolph, "Society," *New York Daily News,* May 4, 1935, Newspapers.com.
9. Mary Margaret McBride, "Noted Decorator Mingles Modern and Antique," *Sheboygan Press,* Sept. 28, 1935, Newspapers.com.

10. Gunther, *Taken at the Flood*, 223.
11. Gunther, *Taken at the Flood*, 233.
12. Gunther, *Taken at the Flood*, 234.
13. "Singer Doris Kenyon Divorces 3d Husband," *Louisville Courier-Journal*, June 9, 1939, Newspapers.com.
14. Corisande, "Older Women Were Loveliest at Holland House," London *Evening Standard*, July 7, 1939, Newspapers.com.
15. "Court and Society," *The Observer*, July 9, 1939.

Chapter 3: "You Don't Need My Kind of Money"

1. John Gunther, *Taken at the Flood: The Story of Albert D. Lasker* (New York: Harper and Brothers, 1960), 174–176.
2. Michael Drury, "Mary Woodard Lasker," *McCall's*, Nov. 1961, 51.
3. Gunther, *Taken at the Flood*, 260.
4. Marvin Moser, "Historical Perspectives on the Management of Hypertension," *Journal of Clinical Hypertension* 8, no. 58 (Aug. 2006): 15–20.
5. Cornelius A. Harper, "Urges Moderation to Cut Cerebral Hemorrhage Toll," *Madison Capital Times*, May 11, 1939, Newspapers.com.
6. B. J. Lockhart, "Mrs. Anna Rosenberg," *Vassar Chronicle*, Feb. 19, 1955.
7. Gunther, *Taken at the Flood*, 287.
8. Gunther, *Taken at the Flood*, 274.
9. Gunther, *Taken at the Flood*, 316.
10. "Speech by Franklin D. Roosevelt, New York (Transcript)," Library of Congress, https://www.loc.gov/resource/afc1986022.afc1986022_ms2201/?st=text.
11. Hedda Hopper, "Hollywood," *New York Daily News*, July 14, 1943, Newspapers .com.
12. Judith Robinson, *Noble Conspirator: Florence S. Mahoney and the Rise of the National Institutes of Health* (Washington, DC: Francis Press, 2001), 52.
13. Richard Malkin, "Digging Deeper," *Opp* [AL] *News*, Dec. 30, 1943, Newspapers .com.

Chapter 4: "We Were the Grassroots Rising"

1. "Col. W. C. Menninger Wins First Lasker Award," *Brooklyn Daily Eagle*, Nov. 9, 1944, Newspapers.com.
2. John Gunther, *Taken at the Flood: The Story of Albert D. Lasker* (New York: Harper and Brothers, 1960), 269–272; Jeffrey L. Cruikshank and Arthus W. Schultz, *The Man Who Sold America: The Amazing (but True!) Story of Albert D. Lasker and the Creation of the Advertising Century* (Boston: Harvard Business Review Press, 2010).
3. Gunther, *Taken at the Flood*, 272.
4. Stephen P. Strickland, *Politics, Science, and Dread Disease: A Short History of United States Medical Research Policy* (Cambridge, MA: Harvard University Press, 1972), 1.
5. Strickland, *Politics, Science, and Dread Disease*, 12–13.
6. Margaret Mara, "Women's Field Army Credited with Fighting Great Fear of Cancer," *Brooklyn Daily Eagle*, Mar. 30, 1945.
7. "Fibber McGee and Molly Radio Show Cancer Special," Apr. 28, 1945, https://www.youtube.com/watch?v=Ep28D0Q1by0.

8. Judith Robinson, *Noble Conspirator: Florence S. Mahoney and the Rise of the National Institutes of Health* (Washington, DC: Francis Press, 2001), 50.

9. U.S. Congress, Senate, Committee on Education and Labor, "A Resolution Authorizing an Investigation of the Educational and Physical Fitness of the Civilian Population as Related to National Defense," 78th Congress, March 1–2, 1944, 204.

10. Gunther, *Taken at the Flood*, 317.

11. Vannevar Bush, "Science: The Endless Frontier," Office of Research and Scientific Development, July 1945, xiii.

12. U.S. Congress, Senate, "A Resolution," 2177.

13. Gunther, *Taken at the Flood*, 307.

Chapter 5: "Money Is Just Frozen Energy"

1. "Unfinished Portrait of Franklin D. Roosevelt," Wikipedia, https://en.wikipedia .org/wiki/Unfinished_portrait_of_Franklin_D._Roosevelt, accessed February 20, 2023.

2. Eleanor Roosevelt, "My Day," *Poughkeepsie Journal*, Nov. 24, 1945, Newspapers .com.

3. AMA Head, "Doctors Fight Regimentation," *Spokane Spokesman Review*, Dec. 4, 1945, Newspapers.com.

4. U.S. Congress, Senate, Committee on Education and Labor, "A Resolution Authorizing an Investigation of the Educational and Physical Fitness of the Civilian Population as Related to National Defense," 78th Congress, March 1–2, 1944, 2031.

5. Judith Robinson, *Noble Conspirator: Florence S. Mahoney and the Rise of the National Institutes of Health* (Washington, DC: Francis Press, 2001), 71.

6. Robinson, *Noble Conspirator*, 54.

7. Lucille Leimert, "Women Urged to Speed Research to Curb Disease," *Los Angeles Times*, Apr. 7, 1946, Newspapers.com.

8. "Veteran Aid Insufficient, Woman Expert Declares," *Los Angeles Times*, Apr. 1, 1946, Newspapers.com.

9. U.S. Congress, House, Subcommittee on Appropriations, Department of Labor, "Federal Security Agency Appropriation Bill for 1947," 79th Congress, 2nd session, May 15, 1946, 291.

Chapter 6: "Can I Help You?"

1. 24/7 Wall St., "How Many People Died the Year You Were Born," June 8, 2020, https://247wallst.com/special-report/2020/06/08/how-many-people-died-the -year-you-were-born-2/3/.

2. Judith Robinson, *Noble Conspirator: Florence S. Mahoney and the Rise of the National Institutes of Health* (Washington, DC: Francis Press, 2001), 102.

3. John Gunther, *Taken at the Flood: The Story of Albert D. Lasker* (New York: Harper and Brothers, 1960), 312.

4. Gunther, *Taken at the Flood*, 333.

5. Gunther, *Taken at the Flood*, 336–337.

6. Gunther, *Taken at the Flood*, 337.

7. Gunther, *Taken at the Flood*, 313.

8. American Cancer Society and the National Cancer Institute, "Facing the Facts About Cancer," 1947.
9. John Kent, "Must Find How Cells Grow to Effect a Cancer Cure," *Olean* (NY) *Times Herald,* Apr. 6, 1950, Newspapers.com.
10. Siddhartha Mukherjee, *The Emperor of All Maladies: A Biography of Cancer* (New York: Scribner, 2010), 18–20.
11. "Leukemia Victims' Life Span Prolonged," *Windsor* (ON) *Star,* Apr. 9, 1948, Newspapers.com.
12. "New Drug Delays Death in Some Leukemia Cases," *Indianapolis Star,* Aug. 26, 1948, Newspapers.com.
13. Sidney Farber et al., "Temporary Remissions in Acute Leukemia in Children Produced by Folic Acid Antagonist, 4-Aminopteroyl-Glutamic Acid (Aminopterin)," *New England Journal of Medicine* 238, no. 23 (1948): 787–793.
14. "Profiles in Science: Mary Lasker," National Library of Medicine, Letter from Joseph Heller, Sept. 15, 1948, https://profiles.nlm.nih.gov/spotlight/tl/catalog /nlm:nlmuid-101584665X141-doc.
15. Gunther, *Taken at the Flood,* 339.
16. Michael Drury, "Mary Woodard Lasker," *McCall's,* Nov. 1961, 51.
17. Gunther, *Taken at the Flood,* 312–314.
18. *Minneapolis Star,* Aug. 14, 1951, Newspapers.com.
19. Earl Wilson, "It Happened Last Night," *Camden* (NJ) *Courier-Post,* Feb. 22, 1952, Newspapers.com.
20. Drury, "Mary Woodard Lasker," 51.

Chapter 7: "We Did It the Hard Way"

1. Michael Drury, "Mary Woodard Lasker," *McCall's,* Nov. 1961, 51.
2. "Freedom of Selection," *Tallahassee Democrat,* June 6, 1952, Newspapers.com.
3. Boris Smolar, "Between You and Me," *Wisconsin Jewish Chronicle,* June 6, 1952, Newspapers.com.
4. Leonard Lyon, "The Lyons Den," *Davenport* (IA) *Quad-City Times,* June 4, 1952, Newspapers.com.
5. John Gunther, *Taken at the Flood: The Story of Albert D. Lasker* (New York: Harper and Brothers, 1960), 331.
6. "Constitution Annotated: Analysis and Interpretation of the U.S. Constitution," https://constitution.congress.gov/browse/essay/artI-S9-C7-1/ALDE_00001095/.
7. "Profiles in Science: John Fogarty," National Library of Medicine, https://profiles .nlm.nih.gov/spotlight/hr/feature/biographical-overview.
8. "Profiles in Science: John Fogarty," National Library of Medicine, Letter to Frank Keefe, Jan. 20, 1951, https://profiles.nlm.nih.gov/spotlight/hr/catalog/nlm:nlmuid -101743404X47-doc.
9. Judith Robinson, *Noble Conspirator: Florence S. Mahoney and the Rise of the National Institutes of Health* (Washington, DC: Francis Press, 2001), 84–85.
10. Bob Considine, "Queen Rises Before Dawn for Coronation Ceremony," *Allentown* (PA) *Morning Call,* June 2, 1953, Newspapers.com.
11. "The Scene Like an Elizabethan Fantasy," *Birmingham Post,* June 3, 1953, Newspapers.com.
12. Drury, "Mary Woodard Lasker," 51.

13. Stephen P. Strickland, *Politics, Science, and Dread Disease: A Short History of United States Medical Research Policy* (Cambridge, MA: Harvard University Press, 1972), 54.
14. Drury, "Mary Woodard Lasker," 51.
15. Drury, "Mary Woodard Lasker," 51.
16. "Profiles in Science: Mike Gorman," National Library of Medicine, https://profiles.nlm.nih.gov/spotlight/tg/feature/biographical-overview.
17. Robinson, *Noble Conspirator*, 35.
18. Strickland, *Politics, Science, and Dread Disease*, 145.
19. Strickland, *Politics, Science, and Dread Disease*, 93.
20. Strickland, *Politics, Science, and Dread Disease*, 150–151.
21. "Bloom," *Syracuse Post-Standard*, Apr. 10, 1960, Newspapers.com.

Chapter 8: "We Thought We'd Have More Time"

1. "Kennedy Opens Candidacy for Demo Nomination," *El Paso Herald-Post*, Jan. 2, 1960, Newspapers.com.
2. Herb Lyon, "Town Ticker," *Chicago Tribune*, Dec. 1, 1959, Newspapers.com.
3. Richard A. Rettig, *Cancer Crusade: The Story of the National Cancer Act of 1971* (New York: Author's Choice Press, 1977), 54.
4. "Profiles in Science: Mary Lasker," National Library of Medicine, Letter from Sidney Farber, Aug. 19, 1955, https://profiles.nlm.nih.gov/spotlight/tl/catalog/nlm:nlmuid-101584665X108-doc.
5. Vincent DeVita Jr. and Edward Chu, "A History of Cancer Chemotherapy," *Cancer Research* 68, no. 21 (Nov. 1, 2008): 8643–8653.
6. Eleanor Lambert, "Lasker Houseparty: Holiday for Friends," *Miami Herald*, Aug. 2, 1964, Newspapers.com
7. "3 Gunmen Loot Jewelry Shop," *Bridgeport Post*, Sept. 26, 1961, Newspapers.com.
8. "Bay of Pigs," Wikipedia, https://en.wikipedia.org/wiki/Bay_of_Pigs, accessed Jan. 4, 2023.
9. U.S. Congress, *Congressional Record*, vol. 140, no. 16, 103rd Congress, Feb. 23, 1994, https://www.govinfo.gov/content/pkg/CREC-1994-02-23/html/CREC-1994-02-23-pt1-PgS20.htm.
10. Thomas Thompson, "The Doctors' Bitter Feud," *Life*, Apr. 10, 1970, 62B–74.
11. "Richard Nixon's Letter to Jackie Kennedy," Richard Nixon Foundation, https://www.nixonfoundation.org/2013/11/richard-nixons-letter-jackie-kennedy/.
12. Robert Caro, *The Years of Lyndon Johnson: The Path to Power* (New York: Alfred A. Knopf, 1982), 275.
13. "Oral History Transcript, Anna Rosenberg Hoffman," interviewed by Joe B. Frantz, LBJ Presidential Library, Nov. 2, 1973, https://www.discoverlbj.org/item/oh-hoffmana-19731102-1-78-61.
14. Julia Sweig, *Lady Bird Johnson: Hiding in Plain Sight* (New York: Random House, 2021), 40.

Chapter 9: "It's Just Piddling"

1. "Person to Person," Media Burn, May 22, 1959, https://mediaburn.org/video/person-to-person/.

2. "The Long War on Cancer," Retro Report, Nov. 4, 2013, https://www.retroreport.org/video/the-long-war-on-cancer/.

3. Stephen P. Strickland, *Politics, Science, and Dread Disease: A Short History of United States Medical Research Policy* (Cambridge, MA: Harvard University Press, 1972), 99.

4. "Cutter Laboratories," Wikipedia, https://en.wikipedia.org/wiki/Cutter_Laboratories, accessed Oct. 5, 2022.

5. Judith Robinson, *Noble Conspirator: Florence S. Mahoney and the Rise of the National Institutes of Health* (Washington, DC: Francis Press, 2001), 114.

6. Strickland, *Politics, Science, and Dread Disease,* 185.

7. James Shannon, "Alan Gregg Memorial Lecture," *Journal of Medical Education* 41, no. 6 (June 1967).

8. Strickland, *Politics, Science, and Dread Disease,* 201.

9. Dennis L. Breo, "The Lasker Awards—Honoring the Spirit of Medical Science," *Journal of the American Medical Association* 266, no. 13 (1991): 1843–1845, doi:10.1001/jama.1991.03470130123044.

10. Breo, "The Lasker Awards," 1843.

11. Frank Cormier, "Johnson Embarks on Poverty Tour," *Dover (OH) Daily Reporter,* Apr. 24, 1964, Newspapers.com.

12. "LBJ Reveals Development Plan," *Lancaster Eagle-Gazette,* May 7, 1964, Newspapers.com.

13. Curt Hanes, "LBJ Appeals for Better Life," *Lansing State Journal,* May 22, 1964, Newspapers.com.

14. Julia Sweig, *Lady Bird Johnson: Hiding in Plain Sight* (New York: Random House, 2021), 40.

15. Frank Cormier, "LBJ Uses Soviet Shift for Campaign Fodder," *Daily Item,* Oct. 16, 1964, Newspapers.com.

16. Marie Ridder, "Capital Revs Up for Party Whirl," *Long Beach* (CA) *Independent,* Jan. 17, 1965, Newspapers.com.

17. "The Johnson Transition," UVA—Miller Center, https://millercenter.org/the-presidency/educational-resources/johnson-transition.

18. C. M. Herring, "Counterinsurgency: An American Journey," MA thesis, University of Arkansas, Fayetteville, 2022, https://scholarworks.uark.edu/etd/4590.

19. "I Feel Like a Jackass . . . ," *The Vietnam War,* Ken Burns and Lynn Novak, producers and directors (2017; Florentine Films, PBS).

20. Telephone conversation #1442, President Johnson to Mary Lasker, Jan. 20, 1964, https://www.discoverlbj.org/item/tel-01442.

21. "President Urges Expansion of Federal Medical Care and Research," *Chicago Tribune,* Feb. 11, 1964, Newspapers.com.

22. Clarence G. Lasby, "The War on Disease," in *The Johnson Years,* volume 2, *Vietnam, the Environment, and Science,* ed. Robert A. Divine (Lawrence: University Press of Kansas, 1987), 189.

23. "Oral History Transcript, Michael E. DeBakey," interviewed by David G. McComb, LBJ Presidential Library, June 29, 1969, https://www.discoverlbj.org/item/oh-debakeym-19690629-1-78-12.

24. "Report to the President: A National Program to Conquer Heart Disease, Cancer and Stroke," December 1964.

25. James McCartney, "$3 Billion War on Cancer, Heart Illness, Stroke Urged," *Minneapolis Star,* Dec. 9, 1964.

Chapter 10: "A Disaster of Such Unparalleled Proportion"

1. Lyndon Johnson, "January 12, 1966: State of the Union," https://millercenter.org/the-presidency/presidential-speeches/january-12-1966-state-union.
2. "Vietnam War Allied Troop Levels 1960–73," https://www.americanwarlibrary.com/vietnam/vwatl.htm.
3. "Cancer Will Take Life Every Two Minutes," *Paterson* (NJ) *News,* Oct. 17, 1966, Newspapers.com.
4. "Lady Bird Johnson's Floral Legacy," White House Historical Association, https://www.whitehousehistory.org/lady-bird-johnsons-floral-legacy.
5. Julia Sweig, *Lady Bird Johnson: Hiding in Plain Sight* (New York: Random House, 2021), 81.
6. "The Beautification Campaign," PBS, https://www.pbs.org/ladybird/shattered dreams/shattereddreams_report.html, accessed Aug. 28, 2002.
7. "The Beautification Campaign."
8. Leonard Lyons, "The Lyons Den," *Buffalo News,* June 17, 1966, Newspapers.com.
9. Robert Young, "Johnson Gets Food Market Study Report," *Chicago Tribune,* June 28, 1966, Newspapers.com.
10. Stephen P. Strickland, *Politics, Science, and Dread Disease: A Short History of United States Medical Research Policy* (Cambridge, MA: Harvard University Press, 1972), 208.
11. "Gains Made in Health Research," *Kansas City Times,* July 22, 1967.
12. "Truman Capote's 'In Cold Blood' Still the Standard," *Chicago Tribune,* Dec. 24, 2005, https://www.chicagotribune.com/news/ct-xpm-2005-12-25-0512240030-story.html.
13. "Bouncing Ball . . . Capote Style," *Rochester* (NY) *Democrat and Chronicle,* Nov. 27, 1966, Newspapers.com.
14. "Party's a Social 'Happening,'" *Tampa Times,* Nov. 28, 1966, Newspapers.com.
15. "Congressman John Fogarty Dies in Office," *Indianapolis Star,* Jan. 11, 1967.
16. "Remarks upon Presenting the Heart-of-the-Year Award to Representative John E. Fogarty," American Presidency Project, Feb. 3, 1966, https://www.presidency.ucsb.edu/documents/remarks-upon-presenting-the-heart-the-year-award-representative-john-e-fogarty.
17. "March 31, 1968: Remarks on Decision Not to Seek Re-Election," UVA—Miller Center, https://millercenter.org/the-presidency/presidential-speeches/march-31-1968-remarks-decision-not-seek-re-election.
18. "Johnson Trails Down Truman's Path," *Binghamton* (NY) *Press and Sun-Bulletin,* Apr. 1, 1968, Newspapers.com.
19. Peter Lisagor, "LBJ's 'Bombshell' Creating Traumas in Both Parties," *Binghamton* (NY) *Press and Sun-Bulletin,* Apr. 1, 1968, Newspapers.com.

Chapter 11: "A Simple Pill That a Simple Physician Can Give to a Suffering Patient"

1. John A. Farrell, *Richard Nixon: The Life* (New York: Vintage Books, 2017), 348.
2. "Inauguration Day Timetable," *Baltimore Sun,* Jan. 20, 1969, Newspapers.com.
3. Carleton B. Chapman, "Flaws in Regional Medical Law Need Ironing Out," *Boston Globe,* Oct. 21, 1967, Newspapers.com.

4. Carl M. Cobb, "'Care for All' Up to Congress," *Boston Globe,* Dec. 17, 1967, Newspapers.com.
5. Gwen Morgan, "Blair, Deeda Wed amid Pomp," *Chicago Tribune,* Sept. 10, 1961, Newspapers.com.
6. Andrew Solomon, "Deeda Blair's Elegance of Conviction," *New York Times Style Magazine,* May 31, 2013.
7. Marie Brenner, "D.C. Classic," *House Beautiful,* Sept. 2001.
8. John L. Moore, "Yarborough 'Mr. Health,'" *San Antonio Express,* Jan. 16, 1969, Newspapers.com.
9. Excerpts from John F. Kennedy's Speech to Congress, "Urgent National Needs," May 25, 1961, Wayback Machine, Internet Archive, "https://web.archive.org/web /20090219141758/http://archives.cnn.com/2001/TECH/space/05/25/kennedy .moon/speech.excerpts.pdf.
10. "Nixon Phone Call," *Binghamton* (NY) *Press and Sun-Bulletin,* July 21, 1969, Newspapers.com.
11. "Formal Charges Filed Against Kennedy," *Palo Alto Peninsula Times Tribune,* July 21, 1969, Newspapers.com.
12. Soloman Garb, *Cure Cancer: A National Goal* (New York: Springer, 1968), 6.
13. Ken Ringle, "Shaken Foundation," *Washington Post,* Apr. 9, 1997.
14. "Profiles in Science: Mary Lasker," National Library of Medicine, Letter from Sidney Farber, Dec. 31, 1969, https://profiles.nlm.nih.gov/spotlight/tl/catalog/nlm :nlmuid-101584665X167-doc.
15. Farrell, *Richard Nixon,* 374.
16. Tim Weiner, *One Man Against the Wind: The Tragedy of Richard Nixon* (New York: St. Martin's Griffin, 2015), 54.
17. Weiner, *One Man Against the Wind,* 46.
18. "Presidential Power—Presidential War in Vietnam," American Foreign Relations, https://www.americanforeignrelations.com/O-W/Presidential-Power-Presidential -war-in-vietnam.html, accessed Sept. 8, 2022.
19. Weiner, *One Man Against the Wind,* 43.
20. Weiner, *One Man Against the Wind,* 57.
21. Michael Dobbs, *King Richard: Nixon and Watergate—An American Tragedy* (New York: Alfred A. Knopf, 2021), 147.
22. "Wyeth Show Opens in White House," *New York Daily News,* Feb. 20, 1970, Newspapers.com.
23. Senator Ralph Yarborough, "Senate Resolution 376—Submission of a Resolution Relating to Cancer Research," *Congressional Record,* 91st Cong., 2nd sess., 1970, part F, 9260–9262.

Chapter 12: "I'm Just a Catalytic Agent"

1. "Profiles in Science: Mary Lasker," National Library of Medicine, Letter from Ralph Yarborough, June 2, 1970, https://profiles.nlm.nih.gov/spotlight/tl/catalog /nlm:nlmuid-101584665X145-doc.
2. "Profiles in Science: Mary Lasker," National Library of Medicine, Letter from Ralph Yarborough, June 2, 1970.
3. Barbara J. Cullison, "Recollections on the War on Cancer," *Science Magazine,* Aug. 21, 1987, 843.

4. "Democratic Study Group," https://en.wikipedia.org/wiki/Democratic _Study_Group.

5. "Oral History Transcript, Thomas Francis 'Mike' Gorman," interviewed by Clarence Lasby, LBJ Presidential Library, June 5, 1985, https://discoverlbj.org /item/oh-gormant-19850605-1-06-40, 56.

6. Richard A. Rettig, *Cancer Crusade: The Story of the National Cancer Act of 1971* (New York: Author's Choice Press, 1977), 78.

7. "Profiles in Science: Mary Lasker," National Library of Medicine, Letter to Leonard Goldenson, Jan. 16, 1952, https://profiles.nlm.nih.gov/spotlight/tl /catalog/nlm:nlmuid-101584665X125-doc.

8. Vincent T. DeVita Jr. and Elizabeth DeVita-Raeburn, *The Death of Cancer* (New York: Sarah Crichton Books, 2015), 118.

9. Rettig, *Cancer Crusade,* 89.

10. Rettig, *Cancer Crusade,* 91.

11. "Profiles in Science: Mary Lasker," National Library of Medicine, Letter from Lister Hill, June 16, 1970, https://profiles.nlm.nih.gov/spotlight/tl/catalog/nlm :nlmuid-101584665X68-doc.

12. "Women Are Nearly Half of U.S. Workforce but Only 27% of STEM Workers," United States Census Bureau, https://www.census.gov/library/stories/2021/01 /women-making-gains-in-stem-occupations-but-still-underrepresented.html, accessed July 8, 2022; "Women Physician PIONEERS of the 1960s: Their Lives and Profession Over a Half Century," https://calendars.library.ucsf.edu /event/8886108, accessed July 8, 2022.

13. "Vietnam War Allied Troop Levels 1960–73," American War Library, https:// www.americanwarlibrary.com/vietnam/vwatl.htm, accessed Sept. 19, 2022.

14. George Gallup, "Backers of Immediate War Withdrawal Rise Sharply," *Honolulu Star-Bulletin,* Feb. 14, 1970, Newspapers.com.

15. Senator Ralph Yarborough, "Senate Resolution 376—Submission of a Resolution Relating to Cancer Research," *Congressional Record,* 91st Cong., 2nd sess., 1970, part F, 9260–9262.

16. Rettig, *Cancer Crusade,* 96.

17. Rettig, *Cancer Crusade,* 99.

18. Jerry E. Bishop, "National Goal: Curing Cancer by 1976," *Wall Street Journal,* Aug. 26, 1970, ProQuest Historical Newspapers.

19. Robert J. Bazell, "Cancer Research: Senate Consultants Likely to Push for Planned Assault," *Science Magazine,* Oct. 16, 1970, 304.

20. Rettig, *Cancer Crusade,* 75.

21. William E. Howard, "Conquest of Cancer Is Group's Goal," *Corpus Christi Caller-Times,* Oct. 25, 1970, Newspapers.com.

22. James Brady, "Wife in the White House," *Chicago Tribune,* Nov. 1, 1970, Newspapers.com.

23. "Lady Bird's Diary Big Seller in Washington," *Ogden Standard-Examiner,* Nov. 1, 1970, Newspapers.com.

24. *Congressional Record,* Proceedings and Debates of the 91st Congress, Second Session, Senate, Dec. 4, 1970, 39944.

25. "Senate Rejects SST Fund, Foes of Plane Jubilant," *Camden* (NJ) *Courier-Post,* Dec. 4, 1970, Newspapers.com.

26. U.S. Congress, Senate, Committee on Labor and Public Welfare, Report of the National Panel of Consultants on the Conquest of Cancer, 91st Congress, 2nd sess., 1970, 4.
27. Report of the National Panel of Consultants on the Conquest of Cancer, 4.
28. Report of the National Panel of Consultants on the Conquest of Cancer, 4.
29. Report of the National Panel of Consultants on the Conquest of Cancer, 7.
30. Rettig, *Cancer Crusade*, 109.
31. Memo from Robert Q. Marston to Assistant Secretary Roger Egeberg, Dec. 8, 1970, procured from the U.S. National Archives and Records Administration, Washington, D.C.
32. "Cancer Study Needs More Money," *Charlotte Observer*, Dec. 14, 1970, Newspapers.com.
33. Judith Randal, "Cancer Authority Proposal Has Questionable Aspect," *Iowa City Press-Citizen*, Dec. 12, 1970, Newspapers.com.
34. Jerry E. Bishop, "National Goal: Curing Cancer by 1976," *Wall Street Journal*, Aug. 26, 1970, ProQuest Historical Newspapers.

Chapter 13: "We Can All Share in the Eventual Glory"

1. Eleanor Lambert, "Mary Lasker Did 'More Good for People,'" *Akron Beacon Journal*, Jan. 4, 1970, Newspapers.com.
2. "What Is Cancer?," *Connellsville* (PA) *Daily Courier*, Apr. 22, 1971, Newspapers.com.
3. Neal Gabler, *Catching the Wind: Edward Kennedy and the Liberal Hour* (New York: Crown, 2021), 614.
4. Gabler, *Catching the Wind*, 641.
5. "Ted Kennedy," Wikipedia, https://en.wikipedia.org/wiki/Ted_Kennedy#1970s, accessed Sept. 17, 2022.
6. Tim Weiner, *One Man Against the Wind: The Tragedy of Richard Nixon* (New York: St. Martin's Griffin, 2015), 137.
7. "Nixon Says Domestic Plans 'Bold,'" *San Bernardino Sun*, Jan. 21, 1971, Newspapers.com.
8. "Annual Message to the Congress on the State of the Union," Jan. 22, 1971, https://www.presidency.ucsb.edu/documents/annual-message-the-congress-the-state-the-union-1.
9. "Annual Message."
10. "President to Ask $100M for Cancer Cure," *New York Daily News*, Jan. 23, 1971, Newspapers.com.
11. "Urges War on Cancer," *Quad-Cities Times*, Jan. 25, 1971, Newspapers.com.
12. Weiner, *One Man Against the Wind*, 658.
13. "The NASA Treatment," *Honolulu Advertiser*, Jan. 27, 1971, Newspapers.com.
14. Mark Bloom, "HQ for Cancer War Is Set Up by Nixon," *New York Daily News*, Feb. 19, 1971, Newspapers.com.
15. Bloom, "HQ for Cancer."
16. Vincent T. DeVita Jr. and Elizabeth DeVita-Raeburn, *The Death of Cancer* (New York: Sarah Crichton Books, 2015), 135.
17. Richard A. Rettig, *Cancer Crusade: The Story of the National Cancer Act of 1971* (New York: Author's Choice Press, 1977), 127–129.

18. "White House Tapes," Richard Nixon Presidential Library, https://www.nixon library.gov/white-house-tapes, accessed Nov. 3, 2022.
19. "Daniel Ellsberg," Wikipedia, https://en.wikipedia.org/wiki/Daniel_Ellsberg #Release_and_publication, accessed Nov. 3, 2022.
20. Stephen P. Strickland, *Politics, Science, and Dread Disease: A Short History of United States Medical Research Policy* (Cambridge, MA: Harvard University Press, 1972), 268.
21. U.S. Congress, Senate, Committee on Labor and Public Welfare, Subcommittee on Health, "To Establish a National Cancer Authority in Order to Conquer Cancer at the Earliest Possible Date," 92nd Cong., 1st sess., 1971, 1–2.
22. "To Establish a National Cancer Authority," 34.
23. "To Establish a National Cancer Authority," 120–123.
24. "To Establish a National Cancer Authority," 194.
25. "To Establish a National Cancer Authority," 200 –201.

Chapter 14: "If Someone Isn't Concerned, Nothing Will Ever Get Done"

1. Robert J. Bazell, "Cancer Research Proposals: New Money, Old Conflicts," *Science Magazine*, Mar. 5, 1971, 877–878.
2. Henry F. Davidson, "Time Ripe for Attack: Cancer Unit Chief," *Wilmington* (DE) *News Journal*, Apr. 2, 1971, Newspapers.com.
3. Ann Landers, "Bill S-34 Gets a Boost from Ann," *Tampa Tribune*, Apr. 2, 1971, Newspapers.com.
4. Stephen P. Strickland, *Politics, Science, and Dread Disease: A Short History of United States Medical Research Policy* (Cambridge, MA: Harvard University Press, 1972), 271.
5. Nixon White House Tapes, April 9, 1971, http://nixontapes.org/emk.html.
6. Neal Gabler, *Catching the Wind: Edward Kennedy and the Liberal Hour* (New York: Crown, 2021), 661–662.
7. Gabler, *Catching the Wind*, 465.
8. U.S. Congress, Senate, Committee on Labor and Public Welfare, Subcommittee on Health, "To Establish a National Cancer Authority in Order to Conquer Cancer at the Earliest Possible Date," 92nd Cong., 1st sess., 1971, 64.
9. James Cavanaugh Memo to Jonathan Moore, Counselor to the Department of Health, Education and Welfare, Apr. 23, 1971, procured from the U.S. National Archives and Records Administration, Washington, DC.
10. James Cavanaugh Memo to Ken Cole, Presidential Aide, Apr. 23, 1971, procured from the Richard Nixon Presidential Library and Museum, Yorba Linda, CA.
11. "Statement by the President," May 11, 1971, procured from the National Archives and Records Administration, Washington, DC.
12. Christine Russell, "The Politics of Cancer," *Washington Post*, Nov. 28, 1971.
13. Richard A. Rettig, *Cancer Crusade: The Story of the National Cancer Act of 1971* (New York: Author's Choice Press, 1977), 185.
14. Rettig, *Cancer Crusade*, 185.
15. "Oral History with James H. Cavanaugh," interviewed by Carole Kolker, National Venture Capital Association, Venture Capital Oral History Project, June 10, 2010.
16. Leroy Goldman Interview, May 5, 2007, Edward M. Kennedy Oral History Project, Miller Center, University of Virginia.
17. Russell, "The Politics of Cancer."

18. "To Establish a National Cancer Authority," 305.
19. Gabler, *Catching the Wind*, 616.
20. Gabler, *Catching the Wind*, 313.
21. "Kennedy, Administration Reach Agreement on Cancer Program," *Arizona Republic*, June 11, 1971, Newspapers.com.
22. "To Establish a National Cancer Authority," 314.
23. "To Establish a National Cancer Authority," 337–341.
24. "To Establish a National Cancer Authority," 403.
25. Nixon White House Tapes, June 13, 1971, http://nixontapes.org/amh.html.
26. "Pentagon Papers," Wikipedia, https://en.wikipedia.org/wiki/Pentagon_Papers#, accessed Nov. 7, 2022.
27. Peter Coutros, "LBJ and 1,400 at Dinner Hear of Gains over Cancer," *New York Daily News*, June 10, 1971, Newspapers.com.
28. Senate Congressional Record Entry, July 7, 1971, 23778.
29. Senate Congressional Record Entry, July 7, 1971, 23788.

Chapter 15: "Putting It on the Shelf"

1. Lawson E. Parker, "Heart Attack Causes Death of Lawmaker Two Hours After Talk," *Fort Lauderdale News*, Dec. 2, 1954.
2. Richard A. Rettig, *Cancer Crusade: The Story of the National Cancer Act of 1971* (New York: Author's Choice Press, 1977), 199.
3. "Rogers Suggests Separate Federal Health Department," *Fort Myers* (FL) *News-Press*, Oct. 2, 1966, Newspapers.com.
4. Rettig, *Cancer Crusade*, 200.
5. Dr. Robert Gallo, interview with the author, June 24, 1921.
6. Rettig, *Cancer Crusade*, 200.
7. Rettig, *Cancer Crusade*, 201.
8. Henry Ginger, "Beautiful People Offer 'Coup de Grace' to Summer," *Tampa Bay Times*, Sept. 6, 1971, Newspapers.com.
9. U.S. Congress, House of Representatives, Committee on State and Foreign Commerce, Subcommittee on Public Health and Environment, "National Cancer Attack Act of 1971," 92nd Cong., 1st sess., 1971, 1.
10. "Duval Slated to Be Top U.S. Doc," *New York Daily News*, May 12, 1971, Newspapers.com.
11. "National Cancer Attack Act," 196.
12. "National Cancer Attack Act," 197.
13. "National Cancer Attack Act," 208–209.
14. "National Cancer Attack Act," 223.
15. "National Cancer Attack Act," 271.
16. "National Cancer Attack Act," 302.
17. "National Cancer Attack Act," 310.
18. "National Cancer Attack Act," 632.
19. Rettig, *Cancer Crusade*, 250.
20. "Rep. Rogers Replies to Cancer Ad," *Miami Herald*, Oct. 13, 1971, Newspapers.com.
21. Clark Hoyt, "Battle Lines Drawn on Independence of Cancer Agency," *Miami Herald*, Oct. 16, 1971, Newspapers.com.
22. "National Cancer Attack Act," 315.

Chapter 16: "The Most Sympathetic President We've Ever Had"

1. "Cancer Politics," *New York Times,* Oct. 20, 1971, Newspapers.com.
2. Ronald Sarro, "Society Denies It Lobbies," *Washington Evening Star,* Oct. 16, 1971.
3. Richard A. Rettig, *Cancer Crusade: The Story of the National Cancer Act of 1971* (New York: Author's Choice Press, 1977), 260.
4. Rettig, *Cancer Crusade,* 261.
5. "Remarks Announcing the Conversion of Fort Detrick, Maryland, to a Center for Cancer Research," Richard Nixon, Oct. 18, 1971, American Presidency Project, https://www.presidency.ucsb.edu/documents/remarks-announcing-the-conversion -fort-detrick-maryland-center-for-cancer-research.
6. Ward Sinclair, "'Disease Lobbies' Are at the Funding," *Wilmington* (DE) *News Journal,* Mar. 9, 1980, Newspapers.com.
7. Lucy Eisenberg, "The Politics of Cancer," *Harper's,* Nov. 1971, 100–104.
8. Rettig, *Cancer Crusade,* 261.
9. U.S. Congress, House of Representatives, Committee on State and Foreign Commerce, "National Cancer Attack Act of 1971," 92nd Cong., 1st sess., 1971, 41.
10. "Cancer Measure Stalled," *Palm Beach Post,* Nov. 4, 1971, Newspapers.com.
11. William Rice, "Nixon to Push for Cancer Agency Despite Setback," *New York Daily News,* Nov. 6, 1971, Newspapers.com.
12. "Profiles in Science: Edward D. Freis," National Library of Medicine, Letter from Richard Nixon, Nov. 30, 1971, https://profiles.nlm.nih.gov/spotlight/xf/catalog /nlm:nlmuid-101584929X17-doc.
13. "Cancer and the Moon," *Johnson City Press,* Apr. 23, 1971, Newspapers.com.
14. Rettig, *Cancer Crusade,* 272.
15. Marquis Childs, "Needed: A Massive Assault on Cancer," *North Hills News Record,* Nov. 6, 1971.
16. "An Open Letter to the Leaders of Mankind," Dec. 3, 1971, procured from the National Archives and Records Administration, Washington, DC.
17. *Congressional Record,* "Proceedings and Debates," Senate, 92nd Cong., 2nd. sess., Dec. 9, 1971, 45837.
18. Bob Wiedrich, "Tower Ticker," *Chicago Tribune,* Jan. 21, 1971, Newspapers.com.
19. "1971 in the Vietnam War," Wikipedia, https://en.wikipedia.org/wiki/1971_in _the_Vietnam_War, accessed Sept. 8, 2022.
20. Rettig, *Cancer Crusade,* 275.
21. Rettig, *Cancer Crusade,* 276.
22. "President Nixon Signs the National Cancer Act," posted by Richard Nixon Foundation, YouTube, https://www.youtube.com/watch?v=lQYfC9kisHw.
23. Leroy Goldman Interview, May 5, 2007, Edward M. Kennedy Oral History Project, Miller Center, University of Virginia.

Chapter 17: "If You Think Research Is Expensive, Try Disease"

1. Bob Considine, "Cancer Victims Get New Hope," *Columbus* (GA) *Ledger-Enquirer,* Dec. 14, 1972, Newspapers.com.
2. "The President's News Conference," Richard Nixon, Jan. 31, 1971, American Presidency Project, https://www.presidency.ucsb.edu/documents/the-presidents -news-conference-86.

3. Stuart Auerbach, "Viruses No Answer for a Cancer Cure," *Newsday* (Nassau ed.), July 25, 1973, Newpapers.com.
4. "Profiles in Science: Mary Lasker," National Library of Medicine, Letter from Frank J. Rauscher Jr., Mar. 18, 1974, https://profiles.nlm.nih.gov/spotlight/tl /catalog/nlm:nlmuid-101584665X144-doc.
5. Jordan Gutterman and Adam Gutterman, Storycorps, Aug. 12, 2012, https:// archive.storycorps.org/interviews/sfb001943/.
6. Jordan Gutterman, interview with author, Nov. 3, 2022.
7. "The Big If in Cancer," *Time*, Mar. 31, 1980.
8. Edwin C. Bearss, *Texas White House, Lyndon B. Johnson* (Santa Fe: National Park Service, 1986), 96.
9. "The Big If."
10. Liz Smith, "The Stars Are Falling All Over the World," *New York Daily News*, Oct. 8, 1981, Newspapers.com.
11. Jordan Gutterman, interview with author, Nov. 3, 2022.
12. "Mary Lasker Lauded at Awards Luncheon," *New York Daily News*, Nov. 21, 1981, Newspapers.com.
13. David France, *How to Survive a Plague: The Story of How Activists and Scientists Tamed AIDS* (New York: Vintage Books, 2016), 41–42.
14. France, *How to Survive a Plague*, 88.
15. Jordan Gutterman, interview with author, Nov. 3, 2022.
16. Terry Lierman, interview with author, July 23, 2021.
17. Terry Lierman, interview with author, July 23, 2021.
18. *Congressional Record*, "Proceedings and Debates," House of Representatives, 98th Cong., 2nd sess., May 3, 1984, 10965.
19. Terry Lierman, interview with author, July 23, 2021.
20. "Remarks," Mary Lasker, Sept. 9, 1984, procured from the National Institutes of Health, Oral History Office.

Epilogue

1. Vincent T. DeVita Jr. and Elizabeth DeVita-Raeburn, *The Death of Cancer* (New York: Sarah Crichton Books, 2015), 124.
2. Jordan Gutterman, interview with author, Nov. 3, 2022.

Bibliography

Bren, Paulina. *The Barbizon: The Hotel that Set Women Free*. New York: Simon and Schuster, 2021.

Caro, Robert A. *The Years of Lyndon Johnson: The Path to Power*. New York: Alfred A. Knopf, 1982.

Cruikshank, Jeffrey L., and Arthur W. Schultz, *The Man Who Sold America: The Amazing (but True!) Story of Albert D. Lasker and the Creation of the Advertising Century*. Boston: Harvard Business Review Press, 2010.

DeVita, Vincent T., Jr., and Elizabeth DeVita-Raeburn. *The Death of Cancer*. New York: Sarah Crichton Books, 2015.

Dobbs, Michael. *King Richard: Nixon and Watergate—An American Tragedy*. New York: Alfred A. Knopf, 2021.

Farrell, John A. *Richard Nixon: The Life*. New York: Vintage Books, 2017.

France, David. *How to Survive a Plague: The Story of How Activists and Scientists Tamed AIDS*. New York: Vintage Books, 2016.

Gabler, Neal. *Catching the Wind: Edward Kennedy and the Liberal Hour*. New York: Crown, 2021.

Gunther, John. *Taken at the Flood: The Story of Albert D. Lasker*. New York: Harper and Brothers, 1960.

Howard, Margo. *Ann Landers in Her Own Words: Personal Letters to Her Daughter*. New York: Warner Books, 2003.

Lasby, Clarence G. "The War on Disease." In *The Johnson Years*, volume 2, *Vietnam, the Environment, and Science*, ed. Robert A. Divine. Lawrence: University Press of Kansas, 1987.

Mukherjee, Siddhartha. *The Emperor of All Maladies: A Biography of Cancer*. New York: Scribner, 2010.

Olson, James S. *Making Cancer History: Disease & Discovery at the University of Texas M. D. Anderson Cancer Center*. Baltimore: Johns Hopkins University Press, 2009.

Rettig, Richard A. *Cancer Crusade: The Story of the National Cancer Act of 1971*. New York: Author's Choice Press, 1977.

Robinson, Judith. *Noble Conspirator: Florence S. Mahoney and the Rise of the National Institutes of Health*. Washington, DC: Francis Press, 2001.

Shylock, Richard H. *American Medical Research Past and Present*. New York: Commonwealth Fund, 1947.

Strickland, Stephen P. *Politics, Science, and Dread Disease: A Short History of United States Medical Research Policy*. Cambridge, MA: Harvard University Press, 1972.

Sweig, Julia. *Lady Bird Johnson: Hiding in Plain Sight*. New York: Random House, 2021.

Weiner, Tim. *One Man Against the Wind: The Tragedy of Richard Nixon*. New York: St. Martin's Griffin, 2015.

Index